I0469138

Alenka Bučer

My Child, Asperger and I

We Are All Special

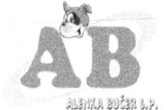

AB

ALENKA BUČER s.p.

Alenka Bučer
My Child, Asperger and I
We Are All Special

Editor:	Alenka Bučer
Graphical design and breaks	Eva Cajnko
Published by	Alenka Bučer
Proofread by	
Print	

For questions and comments regarding the book and published content contact:

Email: **ab.alenka.bucer@gmail.com**

Website: **www.poseben-otrok.si**

The complete contents of the book Being Mother of a Special Child is copyright work and is thus subject to copyright or any other intellectual property protection, allowed only for personal, non-commercial use if not agreed otherwise.

Copying of individual chapters or the whole book without author's written consent is prohibited. Each abuse is prohibited and may result in reimbursement or even criminal liability of the person in breach of copyright.

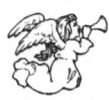

... I am writing this book for you, I want you to know you are not alone ...

This book is a note of a mother's feelings and does not include any professional knowledge and pedagogical actions. It is merely a personal expression of feelings of an adult that was suddenly pushed into the world previously unknown to her.

Alenka Bučer

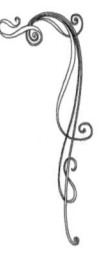

Thank you ...

Marjan Hiti, thank you for all your support.

Rajko Žerovnik, thank you for your help.

Matej Draksler, thank you for being by my side when taking new steps.

Lovro Rozman, Polona Kožlakar, Irena Humek Kok, Erika Trampuš, Rok Cizelj and everyone else who give yourself to others with your heart, thank you.

Marta Pustoslemšek and Igor Turk, an enormous thank you to both of you, your help with searching for the right moves was priceless.

Erin Maureen Grujic, a person with tremendous knowledge, thousand thank-yous.

To the professional team of Šiška Health Center, qualified and warm people, thank you for all the guidelines that lead me to the right path.

Mrs. Tatjana Bizant, Mr. Primož Jurman and the complete professional team of Preska elementary school, thank you for your concern and help.

Topol subsidiary elementary school, thank you for thousand things that are not written in the school rules but are a part of your everyday life and thus worth a million.

Anka Zavašnik and Eva Cajnko, thank you for your help in the process of book-making.

Thanks to Štefka and Robi who have always found a word of support.

Thanks to Medvode Municipality and the mayor Mr. Stanislav Žagar for all the help.

A sincere thank you to all my friends who have been by my side though out those feats.

And thank you, KAJA IN GROM RANCH, your warm people and animals that welcome us, encourage us with warmth and selfless love, stimulate and strengthen everyone that comes to you for knowledge, rest or a moment of peace in this fast pace of life. Darja and Andrej, thank you for each and every positive thought for my children, me or the book, and for the path we walked together and will keep on walking together.

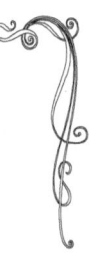

19 February 2008

Regular parent-teacher hours for the first grade of elementary school. This goes for my son, also.

I am sitting tired in front of the teacher, confused from the hard day at work, trying to understand her weird words:

"...your son is very nice, a real sugar, he hugs me when we meet in the morning... He is much better now. I made him a soft bed in the closet; we removed a shelf so he can enjoy his peace and quiet... Yes, sometimes he spends the majority of the lessons there... The only thing is he fights a lot..."

I stare at the teacher speechless, I feel like a stranger that landed on a wrong planet. What? Who is this woman and what is she telling me? What is she trying to say and why am I having trouble accepting her words? This mouth that said 'good morning' so many times before, forms words, I hear them, but deep in my heart I feel I do not want to accept their meaning. Where does my son spend all of his mornings? What is he doing in the closet during the lessons? Why can't he feel safe at his desk, among his fellow pupils? Please, somebody tell me what is going on here ...

I silently leave the classroom and some unfamiliar wrathful mother yells at me with rage, telling me I prolonged the anticipated ten minutes to thirty minutes of parent-teacher conversation, and that everybody has very tight schedules and I have the nerve to take the time that belongs to other parents, and who do I think I am to do something like that ...

I remain seated in the hallway, my world is collapsing. I choke, flames are burning in my chest, I stare into the distance and wait. The shock numbs my body, my intellect is being shut

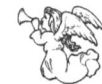

down, my organism blocks all bodily functions and redirects the last drops of blood into my cerebellum. Inhale – exhale – inhale – exhale... the heart is still beating... I am still here. But where am I, really?

I sit and feel nothing; I can no longer hear the hysterical mother. The woman is still opening her mouth and probably spitting out ugly words at me with her grimaces, occasionally even waving her arms, probably trying to present the pain I caused her by prolonging the conversation that collapsed my own self for additional twenty minutes even. I understand her, but I cannot feel her. I don't feel her, I don't feel the surroundings, I don't feel other people around me. I don't even feel myself anymore. I watch her, but I don't see her. I don't hear her, I don't hear children in the hallway, I don't hear the noise from the school hallways. There is only one thing echoing through my head: what is my son doing closed in a closet during the lessons?

"Sucking his thumb" would be the answer of anyone that knows my boy's habits. "Why???" There are at least a thousand questions going through my head and all start with the same word: "Why...?"

Reason and a stream of questions start slowly rising within me. Like a magnet they release numerous words that want to understand the circumstances, define the state of my mind after the shock and through analysis of the past events clarify a new world, still incomprehensible to me.

"Now what? What do I do now, what am I supposed to do?" Only one thing, the moment of this fatal meeting, is filling my brain, numb with shock. One single sentence form the stream of teacher's explanations echoes more and more, all the time. The opinion of a woman who unsuspectingly turned into the epicenter of my concussion is her thought with which I agreed even in this painful moment; my son and I need professional help. But where and how? Why? For what?

"To get a certificate that will confirm that I don't know how to raise children and that my children are really spoiled?"

Those harsh words of my occasionally inexorable reason clear my head in a moment and warm my motherly heart, full of love.

No. It doesn't matter what people think. The only thing that matters now is my child. Trauma of my uncertainty from the past can wait. I want to help my child. I would do anything for him.

"I am ready for anything, as long as I find a way out of this chaos. It is time for me to look for help." This is my decision.

Thus I entered the new world, the world of mothers of special children. This entrance enriched me like nothing else before, it taught me how to appreciate life and accept everything— events, people and children—with all the greatness and love I have in me.

This was the beginning of my new, fuller life.

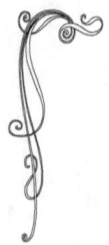

Special or Pampered?

I have two sons, both demanding a lot of attention. It is characteristic to many smart children, but despite the demands they were born and raised with all the love I have in me and with all the knowledge I gained in my life in one or another way. Right after the birth of my first hero I soon discovered that from all the advice, professional or laic I heard up to then, the most valid one is the one carried from one generation to another and I remembered it in such a way: when you don't know how to go on, listen to your heart. Nature gave us all the knowledge we need to continue our species. That is why I follow my heart when the logic fails and then I know I'm on the right path. This is the basis of everything I needed with my younger son for taking such a demanding path to a calm child.

It started with questions prior to testing.

"Date of birth?"

"Was pregnancy ok, nothing particular? Was delivery normal?" they asked.

"How do I know when a delivery isn't normal???" I thought. The fact the professionals ignored at the beginning of tests is that I am not a mother of one thousand two hundred seventeen children but only two.

"Normal???"

Until yesterday I was sure that I am normal, that the school my son goes to is normal, but at this moment I can hardly assert what the word normal should mean to me...

"Yes, there were no major complications," I answered diplomatically. Delivery without complications, child characterized

10

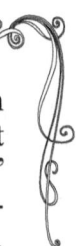

as pretentious; however, all of this seems quite normal with regard to the challenges my life set for me in the past. Most of all, the boy is more normal and lively than all 'normal' girls, dressed in pink, were supposed to be, sitting by the sand-box, listening to their mothers and not getting dirty. Playing, learning with experience and messiness go hand in hand, don't they?

Each birth is something special. Each delivery is different, unique. With both of my sons, when they put the newborns on my stomach, I instantly knew that my feelings were the only right thing in my whole life. It was a feeling with no ambitions, glorious, full of love, perfect in all aspects. I will always be grateful to my oldest son for making a mother out of me. Each moment, I am grateful to my youngest for making me learn how to find myself. But none of that happened over night.

Even though newborns are small and fragile, that wasn't true for my younger child. The moment after the birth, with umbilical cord still attached to me, when they put him into my lap, he snuggled up to me in a very special way. He snuggled to my breasts as if wanting to become one with me, warm and soft, loving and content, as if not coming to this cold strange world full of artificial light and strange hands. His calm eyes were slightly open staring at me, his face in peace, hands firmly grabbing the thumb. In that moment he was stronger than me. I watched him by my side, staring in awe at him and felt his peace as if he was already then trying to say to me: "Don't worry, mom, together we can make it!"

Peace and love were our first bonding.

"Such strong man and already pampered!" the nurses at the maternity ward used to trifle with us. The whole time we spent at the hospital the nurses were competing which of them can cuddle him more. He was smirking and benevolently enjoying each second in their laps. He found love everywhere. He was looking for contact with a person and fed with his peace and love in a totally special way. Even then he was able to get what he wanted. And even then I knew this child was something special.

The way this child became one with my lap, was for sure something special. My son did not hug me. He gave himself completely into the hug. To me, to his brother, to a neighbor or a stranger—once he accepted a person he gave himself to that person completely. To a stranger I was having small talk with at the grocery store, to a colleague I was being nice to because we worked together, or to a friend who came for a short visit; once my boy felt that I trusted a person and that he can trust that person too, he started patting, kissing, hugging, pampering, touching that person ... yes, I was uncomfortable many times, for this trust went too far. He either hugged or spit, kissed or bit, gave all or nothing. There was no middle ground. It was one extreme or another. Both with adults and with the kids he grew up with. His emotions were always very distinctively expressed. Many times his attitude towards his peers or an adult rapidly switched from one extreme to another. At one moment he was hugging a little girl so much he hindered her play and in the next moment he threw stones and sticks at her because the little girl was fed up with the hugs and had pushed him away from her. When we arrived at a playground he 'loved' everybody at first. When we left, he hated every single one of them.

"Nobody likes me! Nobody wants to play with me!!!"

I listened to that every day.

"Mommy, why don't I have any friends?"

I could hardly answer those questions because I myself wasn't familiar with the cause of this over-emotional attitude. For a very long time, I didn't understand what it was that was not right. Are we too emotional within our family? Do I subconsciously teach my children to express such emotions? Do I myself express emotions too intensely? I had put a lot of thought into that.

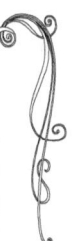

When the boys were little I lived an intense life. Every day, I tried to balance work and motherhood, housekeeping and construction of a house. Many times I just wasn't able to cope with it anymore... Thousands of errands, million things that had to be done, but only one concern—how do I do everything without leaving my children alone for just one moment?

And I don't talk about leaving a three- and a five-year-old home alone and go to the bank. I just wanted to be able to leave a three-year-old with the five-year-old in the living room and go into the bathroom for a moment calmly. It's not that I wouldn't trust the young one with the old one, not at all. The older son was always protective of his brother and in their relationship almost too mature even. Many times it happened that the younger son lost his temper for no particular reason and crashed, broke and threw things around the house, grabbed anything at the reach of his hands and threw things at anyone he saw. During my 2-minute absence it happened many times that I rushed from the bathroom and grabbed the scissors from the boy's hands right before he wanted to throw them into his older brother. I would hide sharp objects from him all the time, but still—when he got upset he did not think rationally. He acted crazy at times like these. He would throw things regardless of how heavy they were and what affect it would have. He would break and smash like crazy regardless of much he loved the person in question. He would repeat that attitude towards his brother, me, grandparents, unfamiliar children in the street or adults he only knew for a minute or his whole life. When he 'lost it', I had to approach him immediately and drag him away from the things that he would send flying across the room, hold him tight and caress him to calm him down.

Similar things happened outside, at the playground among children. Due to such explosions, the trip to the playground became, in his early childhood, very stressful for me. Many times after such outburst the worried parents were angry at me, as if wondering what kind of mother I was! Offensive words that we adults did not hear, of course, would hurt my boy so

13

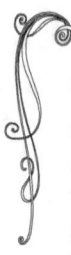

badly that he started to smash things furiously and throw toys around like mad. Children are quick to isolate a peer that is different. They instinctively exclude him from playing and when he tries to blend into the group they often insult him in a really mean manner. Especially, when a visitor returns and his reactions are anticipated by children, they try to trigger them as soon as possible; maybe due to their impatience or their desire to control their territory. The consequence each time was my son's explosion and our withdrawal. Of course, the adults did not make the situation easier in such cases—on the contrary. Aggression among the adult immature population almost always triggered aggression and when that happened I was scared, with my child in my lap and with a great desire to calm down. Only when I calmed down was he able to calm down. I held him tight so that he didn't slip away. I held back the tears and the anger and listened to the stream of insults and harsh advices "what I should do to my child" and "what would happen when they catch him alone." The children's parents immediately became aggressive monsters who threw violent words at us, yelled at me as if I were some spoiled brat that doesn't know how to count to five and is raising a perfect criminal and madman. When parents start to attack, the older children, who are usually the instigators of this hurtful event, almost always laugh somewhere in the background.

Every time, my older son would see and hear everything.

Soon, I started to avoid playgrounds big time. I would observe them from afar, watch the mothers drink coffee and chat about discounts and weather, 'pink little girls' sitting by the sandbox, folding napkins. Each day I'd ask myself what I was doing so differently from them to make coffee and chatting seem so unreachable. But then again I would be satisfied when I told myself that smart children are inquisitive and demanding. I limited my child's company to younger children with which my son got along great and drank my coffee at home with a book or while Bob the builder was on TV. The time spent with my children was still very beautiful.

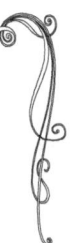

We were too hectic for the society around us. I always believed that a healthy little child had to explore. I raised both of my boys in good faith that nothing is wrong if a child messes his sweater, tears his trousers or forgets his shoes at the playground—as long as he's playing and exploring the world around him. When the younger one made "vents" with scissors into his one-week old pants for the first time because he was hot I explained to him with a firm voice this is not how we do it. In my heart I knew the boy was for sure not stupid. Vents in trousers? An interesting solution. Even when my 'friend' politely asked me not to visit her anymore as they are getting a new Natuzzi sofa I quietly ended my relationship with her. I wasn't able to make my five-year-old and three-year-old sit still for an hour or two to fold napkins with the little girl and dress dolls while the girl's mother and I would praise the beauty and intangibility of her new Natuzzi. The fact that my boys spend more time on the floor than behind a desk was another proof that they are in the phase of exploring. It meant more to me than any sofa, even Natuzzi.

I have to admit that many of my relationships ended this way. My younger researcher was exploring the environment and did not care for all the unwritten rules of the society. Within five years he 'climbed' from being marked as 'vivid' to 'pampered' and then to 'an utterly poorly brought up little villain' in the eyes of the society. During the pre-school period when many of his peers would be staring at a screen for hours I'd cling to the conservative habits and drag my boys outside into the sandbox and put visits to other homes to the lowest level possible. In spite of that we had very good times together. We spent a lot of our time outside, in tents, shelters and all sorts of holes. We were simply together.

It is interesting that many of my sons' peers from daycare would come for a visit. Friends from both of my aspiring children loved to visit us and many times even spent the night at our house. They would jump around the house, chase each other, all muddy and dirty from grass and trees, discover the

15

world around the house for hours. During the whole time of their visit I would be by their side watching that something wouldn't go wrong and the kids would have a great time. At home, on his territory, my son was at ease. He knew what he could expect from the surroundings, he knew all the visitors and everything was as expected. If anything made him angry he came running to my arms, we discussed the problem and then the play peacefully continued. It never crossed my mind the fact that my boy was totally confused in another home could mean anything else than him simply being timid. He was a clever but timid child, a bit pampered. But I did not see the slightest problem in that.

To experience and get to know the world was something beautiful to me and still is. This is what I get to experience every day with my sons. Since the first day of their lives I've been reading to them a lot. Actually, both of my boys were studying my fourth year of university 'study material' as their bedtime story at few months of age and the calm voice of smart words made them fall asleep many a nights. I graduated and we still read encyclopedias together and studied life. I do not remember a day that we didn't read at least one story, a booklet or a chapter from any kind of literature. Whenever the boys got into an argument, got angry or when I simply wanted some peace, I opened a book and they would already lie each by my side and listen to whatever I was reading. Now, they already know how to read themselves but we still spend a lot of time together reading books. Those are our golden moments, our reading and talking time.

The infinite desire for knowledge was brought to our family by my older son already. There are millions of questions pouring out of him daily and sometimes it is really hard to answer them all. The older son likes to ask questions and the younger son memorizes everything. He listens all the time and learns. His memory is like an endless pit. When he explains one of his findings to me, he often leaves me speechless. The boy at nine years of age knows the answers to complicated technical

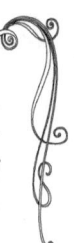

issues and his logic runs like a Swiss watch. There is one more peculiar ability, almost too mature for his age,—he knows how to link events and data into a whole. He even exceeds most of the adults at that and it happens often that we talk at a restaurant and other guests listen. I enjoy sharing knowledge with my boys, even when I realize they are bringing it to the next level, the one I cannot cope with anymore.

What was causing the most problems in our family's everyday life was socialization. Each day we spent on our own brought only beautiful things with it. If I exclude the problems of socializing with unfamiliar people, I have to admit I had only few or almost no problems with my children. They both behave well, especially the younger one. He is more adaptable than most of the children, independent in his discoveries, gentle and loving, and with a lot of empathy. It happened many times that he interrupted his play to bring a stranger a glass of water when he noticed that this person could be thirsty. He took care of an animal, a person or a plant, loved it and pampered it as well as he knew how. But sometimes a stranger would look at him in a very mean manner when my son spontaneously brought him a glass of water or a cookie... If a two-year-old does something nice it is still acceptable to the adults. But when a six-year-old does something nice it is mere self-interest. Is it really? The bravery of a child was many times ill accepted by people due to fear and I felt bad for that. There are many frightened adults and children in the society and I got to know them through my child who offered them his selfless love.

I also found his distinctive independency very interesting. I respected his desire for exploring life in his own, for many, unusual way even if relatives sometimes looked at me strangely. I trusted him and that is why I was able to allow him more than mothers usually allowed children his age. I had an honest talk with him about every issue before an event occurred. I was always careful to present both of them with possible consequences and the decision was almost always theirs. Even if it didn't always seem like that at the playground, I always taught them respect and responsibility and made them aware of the consequences. This is how my older son at the age of twenty months assessed that the child I brought home from maternity hospital was the right one to be his brother (of course I prepared him in advance to all of that) and adopted his decision with so much responsibility that he never showed any signs of jealousy and my younger son adopted an extremely independent way of expressing his views within our family and sometimes left us staring in surprise. Let me tell you about the way my son learned how to walk.

He never allowed anyone to teach him how to walk or hold his hand. He refused any help at learning how to walk from his crawling period on. A young boy, big and strong, was testing movement in his own way from his birth on. When it was time to learn how to walk he would learn hidden in his room when he thought nobody was watching him. He would get up and fall down secretly behind the door of the children's room without shedding a single tear. If I'd peak into the room to see what was making such noise, he'd retreat and pretend to be playing. When he was ten months old, he just came walking one day from his room, independently and sovereignly, and crossed the whole living room without falling once. Of course we were all enthusiastically praising him but he acted like it was no big deal and totally ignored our praise.

"I knew I could do it," was the expression on his face. It was clear to him that he could do it and he accepted it in that way.

"What I am able to do, I can do, and what I can't I don't need it."

His way of thinking and acting was sometimes a real challenge for me if I wanted to lead him through his childhood without damaging his being. He, of course, accepted our praise for his progress, but only for a little while. Then he let us know that he can do anything in one way or another and that life should go on—and the joy had to be over.

He learned many other things in a similar way; independently, in his own way, preferably in the silence of his room, by himself.

While I was around, everything was in order at home as well as in daycare. We spontaneously adjusted our life to a lot of socializing and playing and even more talking. It is still like that now. Many times we talk about life, make physical experiments that are suitable for older children and get to know life around us sometimes in a really mature way. If something is wrong we talk about it, if the children feel injustice or distress I take them in my lap. A talk, a hug and warm words solve anything.

We limited our social life at that time to daycare and home. Both of my children went to the daycare that I carefully picked myself. I still care deeply for their daycare teacher and I have a lot of respect for her. She was able to bring the best out of every child. She is a very calm person and was able to solve problems in the group with love and authority before they even occurred. All the problems in a form of 'explosions' were not expressed in the daycare as they simply didn't occur due to the experience and maturity of the daycare teachers. Another reason for peace in the daycare was also partly because both of my sons went to heterogeneous section with children of different ages from two to five years of age. That is why my son did not have many of his actual peers in the group, especially in the last year. In heterogeneous group, children can learn a lot from each other. The diversity teaches them tolerance towards the younger and the older children and an individual can develop differently. Five-year-olds learn from two-year-olds, three-year-olds learn from older children and I still really like this form of daycare. Today I also know that a child can more easily hide his behavior among younger children in such group that is generally smaller than in classically organized daycare where groups are composed of children of the same

19

age. A smart child that likes to perform and lead the younger children is not a behavior problem; the younger children follow and with his knowledge he is a model to them. Older children behaved well towards my son and because the daycare teachers didn't allow quarrels with provoking words or acts my son never stood out behaviorally. Still more—because the daycare environment was homey to him and he felt safe as he had the support from teachers (an excellent daycare teacher offers support to every child) there simply were no particular problems socializing in the group.

Other than when my son participated at an additional activity and the 'new' teacher saw him as difficult and demanding child I never felt I had serious problems with my child's behavior.

It may seem impossible to someone, but because I limited our socializing to only the inevitable ones in my child's early childhood and we spent a lot of time at home, only us, and avoided the visits, I believed that my son's behavior was normal for a smart, curious child and that essentially we only had to quiet down a little.

My motto that I still stick to was: "He is smart and vulnerable, I love him and I will support him, I will not suppress him!"

I supported my son but forgot about myself...

20

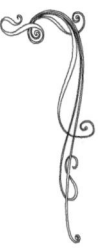

What About Me?

When a woman becomes a mother, she instantly finds herself in a new role. The whirlpool of events at the birth and immediately after it drags her into a world she never really experienced before and the series of new emotions takes her into the new role focusing on her child.

Today I admit: I fell in love with both of my newborns the first moment I smelled, touched and caressed them. I fell in love with my new role at the birth of my first as well as my second child when the first was already home. Each birth was a new experience, unique and one of a kind. Each time I took over the role of a mother with every inch of my being. Only family and work existed in my life. Nothing else.

I subjected everything to my desire of being with the children and building a home for them. I wanted to offer them a beautiful, peaceful childhood and enable them everything. I forgot about myself.

I knew quite a few peers that felt and did almost the same. The first year was quite alright. Three months prior to giving birth to my second child was the first time something went seriously wrong. I felt then already that a demanding child takes a lot of your energy. I asked myself, how I would be able to cope with all of that having two little ones. However, the second birth gave me the energy and I had immense strength, enough for both children, work and the construction of a house. With my devotion to the children I suppressed all my needs even more intensely and adjusted my entire world to the new role. I did not want to hear the reaction of the society.

"My time will come" I used to comfort myself. "I have two little boys. Once they grow up a bit, it will be easier!" I used to say to myself more and more.

Work, home, picking up children from daycare, making dinner, ordering concrete for the house; by the way—all of that with constant watch over my children. Such were my days. I used to hide sharp objects so they wouldn't fly across the room, watched the children play. If there were disputes, I'd hurry and comfort the young one to prevent outbursts and inconvenience after an excitement. I was always there, always with them. I carefully selected moments to quickly hang the laundry and do the necessities in the bathroom and the toilet. Constant planning and organizing became so much a part of me that I was not able to relax even when the children watched a cartoon for ten minutes. I quickly found three necessary chores that are best to be done when I have time! On the outside I might had seemed absent but my system of activities was planned to a detail.

I will never forget a story when I took both of my children to the daycare for the first time right after the maternity leave. The night before I had prepared everything: a small heap of clothes for the older one, a small heap for the younger one, two backpacks with spare clothes, two packs of diapers, and two packs of moist tissues. In the morning, I woke up, fed one boy then another, changed diapers for both of them, put them in their car seats, sat behind the wheel, started the car and— realized I was still in my pajamas.

Many mothers probably go through something similar sometimes; however, it all lasted too long with me. This constant alertness over my children was necessary for far too long and was too intense, too exhausting. When will one child hurt another and with that cause hustling which might end with mad rage of the younger child—this was my constant stress, a threat that was always there somewhere. Just as mothers run after their one-and-a-half-year-old, I'd run after them

22

until school. As soon as my kind-hearted boy approached an unknown child I was in distress because I didn't know if he was going to smack him or caress him. Each play with the peers sooner or later ended in screams and many times I was the one who was scolded at the end. Strangers, family, everyone yelled too many times at me.

People would yell at us: "Spoiled bastard!!!" regardless of where and who was around. If I stood up for myself and for my child the voices would multiply and at the end any ragamuffin that witnessed the event or not would scold me. All of a sudden my university education among the raging group of adults didn't matter anymore and I was being educated by every idiot that met me. In the end, I became too tired and too torn to defend myself; both at the playground and at work.

The worst was with my parents. Even though there are many, far too many people in the society that think they can yell at anyone and educate anyone they meet in the street, those strangers couldn't get to me. I meant nothing to them and they meant nothing to me. It was different with my parents. I was their daughter. At home, the roles within a family are many times mixed up and the rivalry within a family complicates the relationships even more.

Sometimes an advantage but many times a weakness for relationships within my family was the fact that my sister, with whom I get along very nicely, has two girls that are slightly older than my sons. The children get along fine but there is some rivalry between them. It always triggered a safety mechanism in me which was supposed to prevent my boy from having violent outbursts, but then led to such conversations that sometimes made me feel utterly incompetent which can lead to an emotional withdrawal even in the warmest family. Many times in our family everyone was bringing up everyone and each 'well-meant' advice from my mother hurt more than it should; partially because I felt that something was very wrong in my role as a mother and partially because her advices always included me only in a role of her daughter and not as a mature mother of two children. Many times I felt as if I was losing that little bit of authority I believed I had. It was an enchanted circle without a visible end.

What is wrong? Why can't I have a relaxed cup of coffee with my friends? Why do I run after a six-year-old and calm him down in a way suitable for a two-year-old? Why do I not dare to leave him with a babysitter or a neighbor for a short while? Why do I have to listen to all the attacks from strangers day after day? What is happening to me? What is wrong? Thousands of questions drilled my mind every night and the calming words of the daycare teacher, that each child is a bit different just wouldn't do anymore.

New questions would arise constantly.

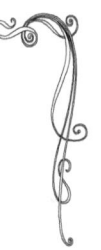

When Singing 'Happy Birthday'
to a Child is Out of the Question

One of the biggest problems for all involved was organizing a birthday party. A special child has fewer friends than other children do and that is why his desire for a big party with many children at his birthday party is so much stronger.

Each year I wanted to make his day really special, just like he wanted. Because he has his birthday during the summer break we celebrated it many times: as a family, then with friends and later in September at school. Each time it was really tough.

It always became complicated when it was time for the cake. At home, we always bring the birthday cake to the table right after lunch when everyone is gathered. Each time we brought it from the 'hideout' my son cried. The distress numbed him so he hid under the table and cried. I comforted him and soon everyone started to sing 'Happy Birthday to you...' but my son started to cry again. He ran away, escaped the hug, stamped, raged and cried. By the time we got to cutting the cake I was exhausted. Regardless of how marvelous his gift was, his birthday went by in stress and less and less guests accepted the invitation. Why does my child experience such a beautiful event that he's looking forward to the whole year in such a strange way?

Another example with a similar kind of stress was vacation. For many years we rented a cottage at the coast. A secure area, in close proximity to the beach and homey furnishings that I was able to decorate myself as it was meant only for us, should offer a nice, relaxing vacation. But it wasn't exactly like that.

The change of environment presented the first stress. Besides the organizational part that is in abundance prior to going on vacation, I always had my hands full with my son. Crying, distress, fear of travel; it was really hard to prepare him to look forward to vacation. Only the third or the fourth trip during the same summer would make the transition to vacation simpler because only then he accepted the fact that we are going on vacation to an environment he is familiar with.

Another big problem was also easy access to the neighboring houses. When our boy was one year old the neighbors understood that he would crawl to their porch while I wasn't around, climb on their sofa, open the cabinets—even then, when they were at the beach or in the town. They even invited him over for some cookies and juice and looked at me strangely wondering why I won't let him stroll around. It is true, the distances between the houses were very short and I could easily watch over him while he was at the neighbors'. But subconsciously I knew that my little boy couldn't tell an sincere kindness from insincere and forced politeness and I didn't know how to tell him that the lady that is alluring him with cookies doesn't really want him for visit because she and her husband are going for a walk. Then already I noticed the boy's naivety and amiability that were later on many times laughingstocks when the other boys would compete who would abuse the naivety of a six-year-old that understands the world as a two-year-old even though he is much smarter than the older kids around him. The older he got the harder it was to hide his individuality and so the expelled child would search for company but always end up as the laughingstock, even by the adults. We were again going in circles; he loved his peers and soon felt mockery, so he soon hated again. It was similar on vacation. Each year, again and again, he was full of love towards the environment, at the end of the season, but after the vacation all family members would mostly look at each other angrily...

Today I understand those events differently. For a child who cannot handle noise and surprises celebrating a birthday presents a lot of stress. A cake is a surprise for a child. Ten children,

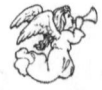

all waiting for a piece of cake, singing 'Happy Birthday' out of their lungs; this is noise. Expecting events brings stress and nervousness. For a child who acts the calmest only in the routine life, there are so many things that indicate anxiety and disturbance and push him into rage and anger. The society cannot comprehend that very easily. Today I know my child wanted company at his birthday party but he was not able to cope with the noise and all the consequences such celebration brings.

Even when I already knew the individuality of child, organizing a celebration for children up to ten years of age was not much simpler. A child's peers expect strictly prescribed behavior at such celebrations and I still have a hard time explaining to them that we celebrate birthdays in a much calmer way, with a lot of games and a cake already cut. It is hard to expect from an average nine-year-old who has almost no contact with peers with individualities to accept deviation from anticipated order of events and behavior at such stiff events as a personal holiday. Sadly, it is sometimes hard to explain that even to an adult.

It is also hard to accept the individuality without negative labels. It was much simpler to drop the lease on the cottage that was supposed to be nice for vacation, adjusted to our needs, than to drop stressful input from the environment. Today, facing such events, I only ask myself what is best and simplest for my child. After all similar experiences my child knows well what a real friend is like and how a real friend accepts your individuality that is why he started to make a selection in his contacts and communication with children by himself already. Only real friends come to his birthday party and this is how it should be.

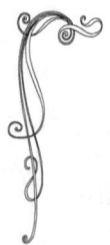

Starting School

In spite of daycare teacher's promises that my son is looking forward to school and that there is no fear of him not coping with the change of environment when starting school, the child's first step into the new system and new environment worried me. By then I knew his fear and anxiety from all that was new well but I comforted myself that the first shock, which was going to daycare, is already behind us and with no major complications so we should be able to conquer visits to school and get used to new order. I completely forgot that this child entered daycare together with his brother and that he had an ally in him in his group so there were fewer complications. I suppressed all worries when an acquaintance—a psychologist—told me that no school can cause serious trauma if everything is alright at home. But still, I visited many schools, even those with special programs. In the end I realized that a child has to enter grammar school and life sooner or later so I persisted in regular form of schooling. I believed and I still believe that it is much better for a child to get used to rivalry and survival in a crowd at a public school right away because keeping your child in a bubble won't prepare him for life.

I spent a lot of time thinking about school when a friend enlisted her child, approximately the same age as my son, to a school with individual program. We talked about the teaching system which was certainly more appropriate for the child. I liked the program but I missed the peers at the school. A child cannot choose a friend in a group of five pupils (the whole school only had five pupils) and socializing with peers at that age is something a child needs the most, in my opinion. Through the whole time of thinking and searching for

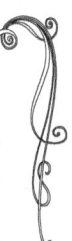

advantages of different kinds of programs something made me return back to the elementary school with generally known program. I knew that I needed professional help and help from staff professionally trained by the state to offer so much help that parents and teachers together teach my child how to live and socialize and do not postpone the problem of socialization for later. Young schools are like young undertakings—they are born and then they disappear quickly, and schooling of a child needs firm basis in experience that only arises from experience through generations. So—due to socializing with the neighbors, due to tradition and preparation of my child for life I decided to go with a traditional elementary school in our vicinity. And I do not regret it one bit.

Unfortunately, I did not know the teacher before the first school day but I did know some of the staff of the selected school and I liked the organization of the institution. The first school day went by calmly. We were excited about the new feat in the sense of child and family development and everything seemed fine. Gradually I introduced a routine school day into our lives and focused on purchase of a house and our move. Together with my children we were looking forward to the new life. My life was beautiful.

But one thing would still bother me. My younger son kept complaining about the change a lot even though going to school was not supposed to be so new anymore.

"I want to go back to daycare. When can I go back to day-care?" More and more often I would hear those words.

At the first parent-teacher meeting I received soothing information that he is smart, that he follows the lessons and that he knows a lot, but sometimes he can be a bit restless and might hustle with other pupils. The teacher's words did not quite sooth me and I attributed it to the change so I talked even more to him. But the anxiety in me kept on going. New Year went by and more and more I would hear he didn't want to go to school anymore. I asked the teacher at the after school care

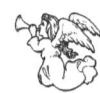

if something was going on, but I never heard anything that would calm me down or upset me for a particular reason. But I had a hunch something was wrong. However, my life was filled up with every day obligations and I gradually convinced myself that time transforms a change into a routine and my child will feel better soon.

On that February day at least a thousand of every day issues went through my head. I found a babysitter for that hour of my absence. She was looking after my children at home so that I could attend the parent-teacher meeting. I cut my obligations to the necessary ones and reserved only ten to fifteen minutes for the parent-teacher meeting because the teacher never mentioned that something could be seriously wrong. I ran into school and there was this hallway in front of the classroom filled with parents with grim looks on their faces. Fine—Slovenes are not really known for generosity towards newcomers. Our family recently moved to this place and I was used to such looks from everywhere else and they did not upset me. Nobody said anything so I sat on a bench and waited for the teacher to call my name.

The room was unpleasant. I worried what was going on at home. I did check the babysitter but she was home alone for the first time with my children and the anxiety came over me so I started walking restlessly up and down and across the hallway, anxious and tense. When the teacher faced me and invited me into the classroom I was already sweating and worrying. All I wanted was to go home as soon as possible. I was mad at myself for letting a stranger take care of my children while I was at a not so important parent-teacher meeting. It would be better to meet the teacher in the morning when my child was safe. But since I was already here I decided to go through with it. In the beginning it was the usual parent-teacher conversation.

"Your son is very smart, maybe a little restless. He knows a lot and has really wide general knowledge; one can tell you

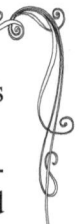

talk to him a lot. He is very emotional, each morning he hugs me when we meet, he really cares for me...!

Yes, this is my son, this is him; his love was nothing surprising to me. The teacher smiled at me politely and I smiled nervously back. In my thoughts, I was still at home with the babysitter so I was not really aware of it when she told me with the same polite smile, that it is much easier now with my son because he has his own corner in the closet in which he retreats when it gets difficult for him.

"We've put a pillow into this corner and removed a shelf so that he feels better now." I will never forget this sentence. It felt like a cold shower in the middle of summer heat.

"For whom did you make the pillowed corner?"

"For your son."

"Where have you made it?"

"Yes, in that closet, where he feels nice." She continued being polite.

"How much time does my son spend in there?"

"Depends on the day. Sometimes through the whole lesson."

At that moment the nice teacher changed into a monster wearing makeup. Everything I anticipated to be wrong just surfaced and everything that made me confused changed from subconscious self-defense into hatred of her because maybe she was unlucky enough to come across a case she wasn't able to handle. Those few sentences were fatal for me. It was not her words that created this turmoil in me. It was my experiences of the last few days and the events that had that same warning sign but I just didn't register them. At that moment I realized that my son was really crying this morning, telling me he didn't want to go to school because a boy is hitting him. I heard myself persuading him that I had to go to work and that we had a meeting and I had to solve some 'work-related' issues. I assured my child that we were going to talk about

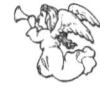

it in the afternoon and that he should bear through that day and then we would look for a solution with which we would both agree.

"Yes, son, just one more day and then I will take you out of school if it is that bad, I promise..."

I felt something was wrong but torn between life and child during the morning rush I didn't know how to save the day other than gaining a few hours with my child. I had no idea how I was going to solve this issue in the evening but I knew I would have to keep my promise. I didn't know to which school I could transfer him and how. My life taught me I can only deal with one problem at a time. And at that moment, my work was prioritized. Now I regret it.

I do not remember how the conversation with the teacher ended. I remember only the awful, overcrowded hallway and a grimaced mother that spit angry words at me with all the disgust an adult could have inside. She was waiving with her arms, yelling and making faces but I couldn't hear her. I was there but at the same time very far away. I sat in that hallway with no air, watching the commotion, as if I were a mini alien. All of a sudden nothing worried me anymore, nothing saddened me, nothing angered. I sat on that bench, silent and without feelings. I vegged out there and waited for something to happen. Something. Anything. Just bring those dreams to an end. Make the nightmare stop. That was the bottom.

When the yelling mother ended her performance, I calmly got up and left. The woman started to yell another octave higher, of course, but it didn't hurt me as I hadn't heard anything. I sat in the car and drove to the next forest. There, I let myself be human. I cried and screamed, I asked myself questions and cursed, then cried my eyes out again. I raged like that for an hour and screamed out everything that came to my mind. What is going on? Why? Why me? Where is this heading? What does life expect from me? What is it that I am doing wrong? What can I do to make it right?

32

The questions were pouring out of me and I knew I had to let it out because my children shouldn't see me like that. I cried and cursed for as long as I felt the pressure in my chest. Somewhere deep inside of me I knew the anxiety had to come out and that I couldn't transfer the fear and the weakness to a child that is not to be blamed. I felt like a helpless child and I did not want my fear and regret of mistakes I had made to confuse my children even more. Slowly I calmed down, suppressed the insecurity with my reason and resigned myself to drive home, although the insecurity didn't go away for quite some time.

At home, there was chaos. The children lay on the stove and the babysitter was hiding in the bathroom in tears. There were signs of tussling and romping all over the living room.

"They are alive and ok. Everything else doesn't matter right now." I felt at ease.

I let the babysitter go, took my children into my lap and calmly asked them as I asked them every day: "What was the most beautiful thing today and what was it that you didn't like? What are we going to remember this beautiful day by?" Talking to them gave me strength again and I knew I had to go on, but on a new path and in a new way. I didn't want to understand. I gave into the moment and wanted to go forward. Instinctively and driven by survival I marched on.

The next day, I took my older son to school, of course, and with my younger son I went to his teacher to tell her he won't be coming to school that day. Another teacher stopped me and started to unveil the curtain for me. There was another boy in the classroom who also just recently moved here and was paving his path in the group of children that continued their common path from the daycare into the first grade. He lived by computer games and challenged the weakest child in the group to prove himself and to be accepted by the group. He chose very cruel tactics known from the computer games when the children were alone.

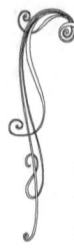

And the teacher cannot be there all the time, right?

With all the everyday chores a person quickly overlooks the obvious. Today I know I should've had a conversation with his teacher a lot sooner. Today I know she also had no idea what was going on because clearly she did not have a lot of experience with children with ASD syndrome (Autism Spectrum Disorder). I was angry at her for softening the problem and for the way how she presented it to me. But as I was learning that children with Asperger Syndrome are really rare and that the schools aren't familiar with the characteristics of children with this disorders I first forgave my own ignorance and then I forgave her. I forgave her the ignorance of individuality and improper attempts to gain authority in the group. Today I admit I subconsciously demanded the same kind of alert control over my child as I practiced at home, which means a hundred percent presence in the classroom, which is impossible, even in the most perfectly organized schools. Deep inside, I maybe even expected her to become like me.

Today, I am aware of all the nonsense and I am grateful that I recognized the mistakes of my expectations of myself, the school, the child and life itself. Now, I am aware that in all that chaos, only a shock that I had to experience was strong enough to help me notice and see and not just expect. I am grateful for everything because I know that the commotion this event caused in our family life created the space for new family basis. Thus we are building our life anew in which only love and peace exist among us.

Thankfully the whole thing surfaced relatively early.

The day after the parent-teacher meeting I transferred my son into the parallel class. With it I rudely pulled him away from his peers but the child's safety was the most important thing for me then. I promised him he would go back to his peers during the after school care, accompanied by his teacher, and the school would make this possible for us. It took him a week to trust me enough again to go calmly to school. His new teacher was a real angel.

My son's trust into school started growing slowly. For the first fortnight in the new class his distress was very big. We spent a lot of time in the morning talking about conquering fear of peers and it soothed him that he was going into the parallel class. His fear was subsiding but it never completely disappeared in this school. Even the next school year when his ex-schoolmate was transferred to another school my son's distress was still noticeable. I knew I would not be able to abolish all the reasons for my son's anxiety. He was at school with more than 500 pupils and it was noisy during the breaks and the noise threw him off track to such extent that later he wasn't able to sit through the lessons. All the impulses that are disturbing for a noise-sensitive child were bothering him. Going to the gym was inducing stress due to the change of rooms. It made the lessons so difficult that one teacher had to stay with him in the classroom. Because of that I was getting more and more afraid of the thought of lessons in higher classes that would take place with the same noise level. Changing classrooms after each lesson and having another teacher for each subject was difficult to accept. It took my son approximately fifteen minutes in the second grade to accept the fact that the subject had changed. His incapability to accept change was so obvious that the teachers had to use pictures with subject characteristics on the blackboard to make him differentiate between mathematics and Slovene language. The teachers also introduced a chart containing smileys that expressed all pupils' feelings. A portion of lessons was reserved for talks about perception, feelings, manners and pupil's feelings if one takes his eraser without asking. My son comprehended the subjects immediately and found repetitions boring and boredom led to teasing the schoolmates or teachers, looking for attention with utterly inappropriate behavior (taking his clothes off, lying on the floor or teasing schoolmates). Such behavior was very stressful for both teachers. However, because they were really calm people, they knew how to establish some trust with him.

35

Gradually his behavior improved although he was never able to sit calmly at his desk through all the lessons. He liked learning and he acquired subjects too rapidly, that is why his boredom wasn't over. Only individual lessons solved this problem, but that was possible only later.

We were lucky that the class my second-grader was attending was calm and quiet, there were no brawlers. The teacher's work with children and especially with my son was fruitful but the progress was slow, too slow for me to hope that my boy could finish elementary school successfully under those circumstances. What am I supposed to do to prepare my child for regular school system? I was seeking for life manual, I read, asked questions but I did not know my way out of this dilemma.

However, the shock was over and it only got better from there. The school organized supervision for the whole time my son spent outside the building, even during the breaks, and the school counseling seriously supported our cause. The social worker immediately called for meetings if necessary and we searched for solutions to the problems. One of the paths led us to a psychologist. This was our first step towards the peace we still enjoy today.

But the path was long. And it started in me.

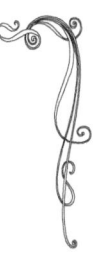

Path to Diagnosis

"My son is smart!" I rushed into the consulting room of a psychologist, who was familiar with tough family situations.

"Of course he is," the wise woman soothed me.

I sat down and she listened to my disconnected sentences that were pouring out of me. The disconnected words, parts of words, interjection after interjection, it all poured out of me and my son was in the room next door, peacefully coloring. The nice lady was listening to me, calmly watching and she politely waited for the storm in me to settle. Afterwards, with my permission, she sat the child calmly next to her and played games with him that clearly served their purpose. Later I called it testing. They were shifting pictures, drawing lines and circles, rotating shapes. I sat aside, went with the flow and waited for the results. The first result of her observations was the evaluation of a confused mother.

"Madam, if you want us to calm down your child, you first need to calm yourself down!" was the constructive criticism of an expert after the testing, in privacy.

"Calm myself down. The woman is not normal," I thought. "I have a very smart child, who, due to his behavior, will not be able to finish school, not even elementary school, and she wants me to observe it calmly???"

The only creature that is worse and more dangerous than a hurt lion is a hurt mother. And that was me. I was hurt, scared, hard on myself for everything that was wrong, blaming myself, my lifestyle and the upbringing of my children. First, I fought with myself.

"They are right; I don't know how to raise children! It serves me right because my job means so much to me! A real mother puts children before work!!"

I was merciless towards me. We are the worst policemen towards ourselves and with such problem I allowed myself to vent—I deformed the image of myself until I was unrecognizable. My being was ruled by fear. During the day I reasonably pushed my feelings back and logically solved problems, and in the evening I played a calm mother, who understands and comprehends everything. At night I was awake with fear, waiting for a new day and forcefully looked for a way out. Each day at a time. I wasted my energy instead of saving it for myself.

The only path that was a shelter and I stuck to it like glue was the testing process. It was led by marvelous experts that were soothing my wounds patiently with their words, and with games and respect towards the child they wrote, drew and held meetings until they separately, each on their own, diagnosed my boy.

My son liked our new days in health centers, filled with games. On Monday, we played with the lady in white gown, on Friday we threw bricks at some other place... The boy calmed down and relaxed outside of school. I heard so many questions each day from all the experts but very little or almost no answers until the diagnosis, they were just sending us from one ordination to another. I cooperated and listened but was still afraid to ask questions.

"He is not spoiled and you are not a bad mother," everyone said. They asked us about our daily routine and I described it, surprised at how well they knew my son's individualities. Each question of a psychologist or logopaedist was oriented into that part of our every day that made my son so different from his peers. Each word that was supposed to be an answer for the therapist opened up a new doubt within me. I know my child, I've been with him since his birth, I feel his every breath—do I really?

Things got better at school also. He grew fond of his new teacher, he played with the daycare teacher and he had nice time with children. When his former class was in after-school care, he joined them often. Slowly he was calming down at home also, but still something wasn't right between us. Somehow, we didn't get along. I was internally restless and subconsciously required more of him, maybe just to show the world that my son truly was smart, but he didn't follow me and he didn't understand me. There were less and less of those silent talks between us. There was less trust in me, less self-confidence in him and less energy in both of us. My fear conquered the reason and the doubt in me grew. Each moment that followed I had less trust in myself and anticipated, through fear, what was going to happen. The day of the results came.

They told me about the Asperger syndrome.

The first few hours after the diagnosis, nothing changed within me or in my behavior. After the mentioned behavioral features and first expert explanations that I listened to but didn't hear due to the shock, I put everything into my subconscious and pretended it meant nothing. I went home with an empty head, played with children and went to bed half-drunk from fear. But the morning after... I can still re-live those moments today. I sat at work behind the computer, a lot of people around me, but I couldn't see them. A morning like every other, everybody was getting their coffee and I sat in front of a black screen. I stared at the darkness but didn't see anything. Asperger syndrome? What does this mean? What now? Does this mean my child is really ok? What does it change essentially? Why do I feel better? Am I less anxious because the diagnosis has a name? The tears of relief stream down my face. Minutes go by, the dark screen doesn't come to life and the tears keep on running. My cheeks are wet with tears of relief, mixed with fear, but the nervousness is gone. The fear of the unknown is gone. It's been sixteen hours since the doctors started offering answers but only now do I feel that I am entering a new world. What now? Will I be learning how to talk to my child? What is it again, that I don't know? The child doesn't understand me—he doesn't comprehend my words. How can it be that a smart child like him doesn't understand his mother? That he cannot understand complex orders? How come? How can a child understand Slovene but doesn't understand the words he grew up with? We do talk a lot more than in other families... What do I do now?

I stared at the dark screen for a long time when a colleague came by.

"Alenka, come to my office, please," he woke me up from the numbness. "Only a child-related problem can crush a person like that. I have a meeting now. Please, stay in my office for as long as you need to, just pull yourself together. Tomorrow after lunch come to my house, we'll talk."

This was one of the biggest turning points in my life. I started to realize then, that I was entering a new world, the world that is different not just by the way of thinking but it has its own language and much deeper feelings. The world that the experts call the world of children with special needs. The fact that I wasn't alone anymore gave me strength. The colleague that approached me was the first in the series of new faces of wonderful people, but, an experience is an experience and the hand that one offers to me today is worth gold. I am not alone. This is the feeling that helped me survive then. There are so many of us, learning mothers. The first thing I really needed was the feeling of belonging.

But how do we go on?

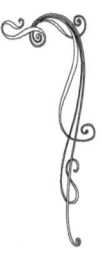

First, the Mother is 'Put Together'

"I can do it and I will do it!" was my motto at first. I suppressed my feelings, put the rein on my life in the hands of my reason and did everything the teachers and experts expected of me. My work demanded a lot of energy, the tests took a lot of my time each week and I spent the rest of my time with my sons. At night I was housekeeping, maintaining the house, preparing plans for our move, selecting hardwood floor for the house... I worked from morning and burned the midnight oil. I read and learned about the Asperger syndrome each evening and late into the night and those last two hours of the night that I really should spend in bed I searched the internet for everything that was written about the upbringing of a child. Somewhere deep inside I was still blaming myself for not bringing my children up the right way and because I had been taught at the faculty that I could do anything with the help of books I clung to it in every possible way. I acted like a student that fails a very important exam—yes, I have to do it, I have to pass the test of 'being a mother'!

But there was no test. There was a day, and then there was another and each was full of new situations. At the health center they nicely told me to keep all the commands intended for my son simple and that I should pay attention to all the specific things he was going to show by himself. They didn't live with me, though, to tell me what was right and what was wrong with each situation. And above all, they never told me how to accept the new role in the new world, the role of a mother of a child with special needs. The label itself, 'a child with special needs', scared me because I subconsciously imagined all the clichés of being special that the society usually doesn't

41

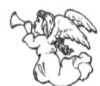

understand. Of course I knew that my son was a very smart child and all the tests confirmed it, but the labels that we subconsciously create and adopt for life are hard to get rid of, especially when we feel that not everything is like we expect it to be or as it should be. For the society, 'special' is mostly related to being mentally challenged and that angered me.

I was also disturbed by all the new questions of the people close to me. I don't know why, but many who knew my family, wanted to prove to me with counterarguments that I was wrong, that the health system was wrong, that the school was wrong, in short, that everyone was wrong. They asked me things I wasn't familiar with and I didn't know many of the answers to those questions. And the same people that were earlier yelling at me that the child is too pampered were now trying to persuade me that I was dramatizing and that I should stop cuddling my child. Many an upright men from my surroundings claimed that I was complicating my life and the life of my child because all that my boy needed was two spanks on his behind. I was torn again. In my desire to find answers I put myself into the role of an observer. I wanted to see how we function in society; how the society accepts me and my sons even, after so many years of withdrawal.

One Saturday in June, about three months after the diagnosis, I accepted a friend's invitation to a firefighter fest. This man seemed open enough, highly educated and reasonable so I accepted the invitation to an event that might make my boys happy. It was a nice sunny day.

During the official part of awarding the recognitions to the firefighters my boys were climbing onto an army vehicle parked in the vicinity for promotion of the Slovenian army. My friend joined us a bit later. He invited the children for ice cream, then some juice and cevapcici. We were sitting in a tent where the music was playing. The younger son soon became restless. He started moving from one foot to another, looking restlessly around and pulling my sleeve, then my shirt;

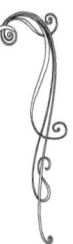

he behaved strangely. He couldn't tell me what was wrong, but I wasn't confused by his unrest because the people at the health center explained some of the most important issues that I should pay attention to. Soon it became clear to me what was bothering my child. Dark, breezy tent, many new faces, noise behind the stage, all of that made his unrest only stronger. When they brought cevapcici, they accidentally put mustard and ajvar together and he lost it. He hid under the bench in a corner where nothing could reach him. That was new and unusual. I persuaded him to come to my lap and my friend brought another portion of cevapcici. But it was too late for him. His threshold was exceeded.

My friend politely said goodbye.

As soon as we left the tent, everything was fine. I stayed at the fest for another two hours with my boys. We were at a bright area, away from the noise and my son played and acted his age. Soon it became clear to me what is it that is too disturbing for my child. I started to learn from him. And that was it. I was learning to understand him.

However, I was still very tough and too demanding towards myself. I asserted that I can do a lot more than I was truly being able to comprehend, do or learn. I worked practically twenty-four hours a day. I pushed myself to the limits of exhaustion, I cleaned and worked, I escaped into work, learning and errands, I planned and thought until I suddenly found myself utterly exhausted in an ambulance. Running away from myself brought me so far that I just collapsed on an ordinary autumn day at work and an ambulance took me straight from work to the health center and then home—with a diagnosis of complete exhaustion. At that point everything 'fell down'. My batteries were totally empty. At home, I practically slept for seven days and seven nights straight. I forced myself to be awake for an hour each day to talk to my children and slept through the rest. I hadn't been so fast asleep since my first pregnancy. Immediately after that sleeping week I decided:

it is my turn now. The time has finally come to put myself in order. Then it was time to find my place in that new world I was getting to know. The moment arrived which I could dedicate only to myself.

When I rested I decided that I would focus on myself. I felt that all the threads were in my hands and I decided to get to the bottom of my fears. I wanted to calm myself down more than anything. On a warm winter day, I went to the near-by forest like I always do when I look for peace.

In the forest behind our house there is a large stump. I call it 'my stump of little angels'. It heard many stories and absorbed many tears. I visit it with my dog almost every day and that afternoon my faithful dog turned towards it, towards the stump. As many times before I sat on it and told him my story of that day and sang my song. I stared into the distance and sang a song of questions and life from my heart. The dog was lying at my feet and put his head onto my lap and listened. And all of a sudden—silence. I hushed and the forest hushed. There was no breeze among the thick trees, the birds were silently sitting on the branches and waiting. The forest was wrapped in silence. I felt my unease.

Then, a stream of screams started to pour out of my throat. Horror, fear and all the past anxieties came out. I was writhing my body and screaming from the depth of my body, yelling and shouting the sentences of horror and fear, pouring the requests out of helplessness and humbleness towards life. All that came upon me during the past months came out and I cried as if I wanted to cry out all the sorrows I had kept within for so long. I had so much woe in me that the raging and the requests couldn't come to an end.

"What am I so afraid of?" I heard a whisper in my heart.

"Ignorance... my own expectations... myself..."

"Life, please, help my child go at least through elementary school, please!"

That scream broke me. I sat next to the stump, leaned on it

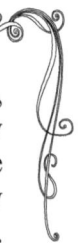

and cried. At that moment I was a small child of the universe, I was a learning little girl in a tough school of life, weak in my ignorance and doubts, fearful. I felt lonely but I wasn't alone there. In that moment of loneliness I felt a dog's snout on my shoulder. He was looking at me faithfully, this dog of mine. He winked at me and kindly put his head against my neck as if trying to sit into my lap. His warmth made me feel safe and soon I calmed down. I cleared my thoughts and listened to the forest's song. I felt much better. I straightened my back, wiped the tears and focused my sight. In a way this forest offered shelter with his greatness, I didn't feel lonely anymore. I felt all those animals that were watching us and there was my best friend, he, who loyally accepts me and doesn't judge me, doesn't ask questions. His loyal look gave me new strength. I felt a new miracle of life next to me. It was a moment of total surrender.

Then I looked into the sky and in my thoughts I handed the steering wheel of my life over to the force that creates the events outside my abilities and expectations.

"Let life go its way. Now, I accept everything and follow life," was my decision. A huge burden of responsibility was lifted from my shoulders. I felt that I do not have to carry all the weight of my family's life. I handed it over to life itself, accepted everything that is unpredictable in life and then I started to breathe more calmly. After that it was much easier for me. For the first time I felt true peace within me. Finally.

Then a cuckoo cuckooed three times.

Exhausted I took a nap by the stump and woke up about an hour later. That day I let go of all my desires and expectations regarding my children and engaged myself to accepting everything life brings me. In that decisive moment of peace I decided to go with my children through everything that is awaiting us in life. At that moment I accepted my life in its entirety.

By accepting all the emotions, events, feelings and lives of

45

children, which is basically everything that life might bring, my life started to calm down. I was on sick leave for a month and a half trying to find the time to find a really suitable babysitter for my sons for my one evening hour of badminton which helps me release the valves. I hired a housekeeper to take over a part of the chores and canceled all the afternoon activities after the after-school care for my children. We found activities during the after-school care that they both enjoyed and we spent the time after work together. All in all, during the month and a half I calmed down a lot and settled my life. Since then, I love coming home even more because peace, hugs, love and happiness await us there. Our talks that were frequent before still fulfill our peace. Acceptance, beauty and love. And peace. Wrinkled clothes on a pile waiting for ironing and long grass around the house no longer disturb me. Of course I am going to do all that but only then when it's time to do it and no sooner.

All that peace within me and within my family was possible only then when I accepted everything that was new and so very unusual to me. I immediately loved and accepted my children when they were born. I respect them and love them immensely just the way they are. I only needed time to accept myself as a mother. Both times when I was pregnant I fell into the whirlpool of sequences dictated to a future mother by the society. If it were dictated only by nature, it would give me peace and time to get to know my new role. Society took my peace and time and exchanged it with twelve magazines, two hundred books and thousands of commercials, in short, everything that was supposed to be the best for a child. University taught me that I can do anything, society was convincing me that the nature already gave me everything and I only needed to select the safest stroller and the best diapers. I only recognized the absurdity during my sick leave when I was able to be alone with myself and my children for the first time.

My lesson was to calm myself down and accept everything that life offers in the exact same form as it is offered. It didn't

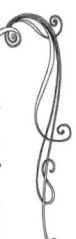

matter how smart my son was. It only mattered that I accepted his individuality also in his relationship towards the society. I had to accept the fact that my child cannot stand noise nor mustard mixed with ajvar and that it doesn't matter what anyone thinks of it. It was important to truly understand that I had to teach him that when I said 'dinner', it mean that he had to stop playing, put away the bricks, wash his hands and sit at the table. Four commands instead of one. Cutting commands to less complex operations is what they had been telling me at the health centers.

I also have to accept that there are children (and my child among them) who do not understand sentences with figurative meaning and that cannot tell exaggeration and lies from everyday clichés. When a five-year-old asked me to explain how the neighbor was actually going to drink the whole lakes and if that was really possible, I was convinced that he was teasing me. Today I teach him that if I say his nose is as big as Himalaya, it doesn't really have that meaning. True, we still talk about the lies that we've set as true in the everyday conversations and it is really interesting to hear those phrases we hear and say every day through my son's ears (which is in its literal meaning also impossible, right?).

Are we even aware of the everyday insincerity and nonsense we say? It is a big problem if a child doesn't understand that. And that problem becomes soluble only when you truly know it.

For many years my son didn't understand me and for many years I didn't know that we just don't speak the same language. Now, that we cut complex commands to simple ones, I realize that my boy is really well-behaved, smart and accurate. Now that I know that even when we talk every day there still is a possibility that we don't understand each other about a certain issue and I accept myself and him more than ever before.

That was a school for me, an elementary school for starting to calm my child down in society also.

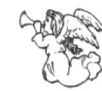

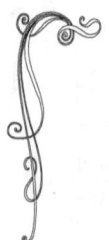

What About School?

After switching classes, the fear in my son's eyes slowly ceased. I still cannot say he loved going to school but the rebellion and the anxiety were not as present as they were before. On a daily basis I talked to everybody who was in contact with him, summed up all the information, looked for solutions, all with one wish—to make him feel better at school. The school experts also participated in those talks and through the whole process of testing and recognitions I was in an intense contact with the school. Until the end of the first grade all of my efforts were aimed at one goal: to give the child back the feeling of security at school. With the help of school we succeeded to some extent. But having twenty-two children in one classroom did not allow the teacher to dedicate more intensely to communication and relationships among children that is why the quarrels were still present. However, the children were under surveillance all the time and the adults were able to intervene fast if a quarrel started and my child was less distressed.

However, it was still difficult for the boy to sit still at the desk for the whole 45 minutes, the duration of one lesson. In spite of the teacher's every day effort it was almost impossible to follow the lesson calmly. There were a lot of exciting impulses in the classroom that bothered the child all the time. He would get up during the lessons, walk across the classroom, argue with schoolmates over crayons and erasers, and interrupt the lessons. After twenty-five minutes when his level of concentration dropped another teacher focused all of her attention to my son to make the lessons at least somewhat less interrupted. Gym and music lessons were many times practically impossible due to the noise my child couldn't handle.

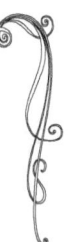

All the love and all the effort the teachers put into their work with children in the classroom with the desire to give my son back the trust into the school and bring the situation in the classroom back to normal were not enough precisely due to all the elements that disturbed a sensitive child every day. Although it sort of worked at the lower grades I couldn't imagine the higher grades in such an organization and with such problems. Something urgently had to be changed before the transfer to the higher grades.

We were all gradually learning through the relationships between children and reactions to them. All of the teaching staff that were in daily contact with my son read all the technical literature that was available on Asperger syndrome. Many attended seminars on this subject. They were very adaptable, nice, and patient; they were just what I needed at that time. I was really lucky that within half a year a group of three experts formed and they helped me find a way out of this distress. A group of experts, friendly school ready to help at any time and many new friends with similar problems that I had was my world that formed an everlasting source of information and directions and all of that led to the root of the problem and to the reason for my child's distress and this to the path that led me towards problem solving. I found my way to the essence of the problem and it all became much easier for me. I wanted to gain more knowledge, know-how, I wanted to get to know my child from the side I only started to notice with him and was learning from it.

Yes, it sounds strange. When my son reached the age of six, I slowly started to realize that I didn't know him at all. Through his entire childhood I've been talking to him a lot on daily basis, spending a lot of time with him; however, in the first grade of elementary school, I realized how much I still needed to learn about him. It was a shocking revelation that many mothers might experience.

For you to understand the individuality and problems

regarding my son, I would like to explain a situation by providing a much simpler example: your child cannot see the color orange. Not only that—through his eyes the color orange is fluorescent and shining and so disturbing that he becomes anxious every time he sees it. In the worst case scenario he starts to rage, he goes mad and becomes socially unacceptable. But you don't know that, you are not familiar with such problems. At the age of three the psychologist confirmed that your child sees all the basic colors and that he is very smart and healthy. Throughout his development you rely on her report; however, you are aware that there is a problem. Your child cannot explain the problem to you because he does not know the color orange in the same way we do! What can you do in such a case? How do you recognize a problem? Where do we come across the color orange? How many girls wear orange every day at school? What can you do in such a case? Our case is similar but much more complex.

Mrs. Erin Maureen Grujic from Maribor told me what disturbed my son. I attended a music camp led by Mrs. Maja, an expert from Center for Autism, and she told me that an expert on working with children with Asperger syndrome lives in Maribor and she worked in schools abroad with children with this diagnosis. After the whole day of testing (playing, of course) she gave me a precise report on my son's abilities and limitations. She proved to me that one of my child's individualities is that he cannot perceive touch accurately. His brain is not processing and making sense of touch to know if touch is pleasant or harmful and so he doesn't know how to react to touch. He cannot feel the exact location of a touch and cannot define where somebody touched him. I was shocked. Is that even possible? My child has been using his arms for six years but he doesn't feel them in the same way other children do? Is this the reason why he cannot tell when his arm caresses someone or slaps him?

We received many solid measures, accurate evaluations and much focused suggestions for play from Mrs. Erin Maureen

Grujic. She provided a lot of advices and suggestions on how to observe, learn and work, which I benefitted from in actual life situations. She taught me how to teach my son feel all parts of his body and which games will enable us to do that as soon as possible. From there on everything was just getting easier. I realized how and what the child feels, to what extent something disturbs him, what bothers him and how he expresses it. This expert assessed and graphically presented everything that I previously anticipated. Finally, the reasonable part of my being was able to understand the problem.

We left Maribor tired but full of ideas on how to go on. The instructions were phenomenal: wrap him in a blanket, play Pancakes to make him aware of the touch gradually... We received a lot of advices and we used many of them. I forwarded the report to our school and I realized that this school was not going to be the right one for him at the higher grades because of the noise and hourly classroom switches. Mrs. Rotovnik, a social worker from Šiška Health Center, had a brilliant idea at the right moment—Topol subsidiary elementary school was much more suitable for my child. This was the right path towards calm environment for my child. In a few months, all people that knew the child agreed that transferring him to Topol was the right decision.

Only—how to explain that to a child that gets disturbed just by thinking about a change, nevertheless the act itself?

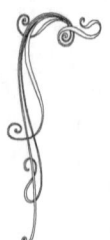

The New Environment

The decision of transferring the child to a new school was carefully considered because the change of the environment causes the most frustrations for my son. Another school meant a drastic change of environment, friends, teachers and everything that was familiar to the child. The boy was in the second grade and I knew that due to the marks it was high time to make the decision of transferring the child or not; that is why I was continuously and systematically collecting information on all possible options at both schools. But every time that I just for a moment remembered the lessons at the higher grades and the constant swapping of faces and classrooms it was clear to me that the boy couldn't stay in such a large school. In the second grade, a third teacher was teaching his class English in a classroom at the other end of school and both teachers of the class that my son visited had their hands full with him. The change was too big, the transfer many times unsuccessful. The noise, the hallway, bustle of children and another classroom— the transition to a new classroom during the break just wasn't possible, no way. They tried to introduce the change during the whole year but were unsuccessful. A hallway full of children represented horror and fear for my son. It represented everything that upset him, all at once—the anxiety due to the crowd, the dread due to the noise, the fear of too many impulses, all at the same time. A hallway full of children was the one thing we weren't able to adjust to or change. That is why I decided to transfer my son to another, smaller school.

At the new school I first met with the management and expert staff. They all welcomed me very nicely. All of the teachers introduced themselves and we had many talks and meetings. Three months prior to transferring I took my child

52

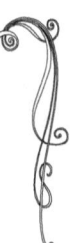

into the new environment for a whole day. Future schoolmates welcomed him warmly and calmly and they spent a beautiful natural science day. On the first day, my child was naturally against the transfer because everything was new to him. He complained among others about lunch which was not exactly what he was used to. However, going back to a noisy school was a trigger for his initiative to transfer to another school. So on 1 September I took my younger child to the third grade at the Topol subsidiary elementary school.

Topol elementary school is a peaceful school in the country, a nine-year program school with sixteen pupils and five teachers under the wings of a strong central school, Preska elementary school, with the support of even stronger professionals and with everything a curriculum requires. Everything is organized and executed in a very calm, nature friendly manner. It is not a small, new private school, dependent on a handful of people that can be crushed by a car accident of the school manager. Topol elementary school is a small world within a large institution that assures personal approach and preparation for regular high school for the whole nine years, taking every child's individuality into consideration and adjusting all of his individualities to the basic social life. That was what I was looking for. That was the most I could offer to my child.

And thankfully—it was near our home.

The school management organized itself immediately after the transfer of the child in a way that all the teachers informed themselves very precisely about working with children with Asperger syndrome. They organized morning care in a school nearest to our home, someone escorting him on the bus to Topol, special teacher help during the lessons, care, help with tasks and attendance in the after-school care until my arrival. The child received his own corner in school, his 'calm-down tent', an escort and everything he needed. The school provided him a laptop to write tests in case writing would hinder his expressing (he was weak at graphomotorics). The school management and teaching personnel enabled everything they could for a child with special needs. They organized a visit and counseling of Mrs. Erin Maureen Grujic, who knew the particularities and special needs of my child very well. Based on her experience she informed the teaching staff how to continue with their work. The child was visibly progressing each day with help of massage, meditation and touch therapy. He was slowly calming down, his self-confidence grew, he was expressing more and more of everything known to him and finally his very positive characteristics were expressed. In a few months my son became a calm child with 'socially acceptable behavior' and with individualities that were now being expressed with high level of knowledge, abilities and sense for art and with abilities I rarely see in other children. In new school his being was expressed.

Today I am confident that not only people make the Topol school so excellent. Through all the tests in all the schools and institutions I collaborated with wonderful people, experts, who focused all their knowledge, feelings and abilities into helping a child. Today I believe that each school is full of such people. All pedagogues, social workers, and everyone working in schools are there with a desire to offer children the best to prepare them for life. Giving a child what he needs takes a lot of their energy. The major difference between schools is what a school as an institution can offer to a child. If a child needs more movement, he needs a school with a big gym and with variety of sport activities in the after-school care. If a child is easily upset by the noise, he needs a smaller, calmer school with fewer pupils. It makes sense that a large school cannot offer peace and quiet during the breaks and that a small school cannot offer hundreds of activities. It is for us parents to find such a school that will enable our child to express his being. I am very fortunate that I can offer my children both: to the older one sports and to the younger one peace and quiet. Thus they can both grow up into calm, creative, satisfied people and learn life in a proper manner. At home I can combine both in my tight embrace in my lap.

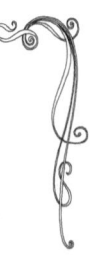

Show Me Your School Report

At the end of the second grade I was surprised by the desire of my relatives for my sons to show their school reports at the end of the school year.

"NO!" was my spontaneous answer.

"Why not?" they continued.

It was the first time I consciously stood up for myself in front of the relatives. My first reaction was spontaneous and I was slightly offended.

"Not once had they taken my children to school or looked after them for an hour and now they want to comment on their effort? Why and what gives them the right to do that?"

Their request or almost a demand upset me. The reason was not that they hadn't shown any interest in them. It bothered me that they requested the insight into their reports without ever really trying to understand. I felt like somebody was trying to compare the hundred-meter running results of a disabled person with the results of a sprinter that trains every day. It is not that I considered my son a disabled person, not at all. It truly upset me when children were labeled and classified by persons who didn't know them well or didn't know them at all and it still bothers me today. It doesn't matter who the child is that someone is trying to evaluate with numbers—each child is a unique, extraordinary being, full of unimaginable potential in areas the assessor maybe isn't even familiar with. The fact that the assessor has read two books on children with special needs doesn't mean that he accepts the child as a whole and any evaluation of such child can only be unjust.

After all, even I didn't know my child well enough and I was aware of it every single moment.

Soon I realized that I wasn't really angry at the relatives. People act stereotypically, just like they have been taught by the society. It was clear to me that they didn't think about their requests; today not many people think about what they do or say. But I do know that I acted the right way.

I support assessment of child's knowledge with numbers, but only within a system, required by school. The fact that a child can through an assessment compare his knowledge with his schoolmates within the same class stimulates the child to work hard and to form work habits needed for life through learning. In my comprehension, daycare is also included into the school system because this is when children begin to learn to cohabitate and they learn the basics of socialization in the sense of schooling. Assessment within a homogenous group is important for us to recognize a child's individuality and to upgrade it suitably. When these children grow up, the society will assess their work and abilities through payment and this is the life of an adult, this is what we raise our children for.

I am sure that if my younger son went to a daycare group of children the same age, his individuality would be noticed sooner. A daycare teacher who has with her work far more freedom than a teacher would be able to notice the child's individuality sooner and the transition to more intense and more suitable work in the field of socialization would be far less stressful for the child and his surroundings. Assessment of a child in a group of his peers would be very helpful. I would be able to take the child to specialists sooner and I would be able to start teaching him in a more appropriate way sooner.

Similar goes for school. The marks inform the parent of what suits a child and what does not. Such assessment can help the parents to direct the child either into natural or social sciences, and later to an appropriate vocation. If we exclude the trend of economists, I am sure that by more realistic view of children's marks many adults would direct their teenagers into a socially less popular vocation in which their child would feel happier and fulfilled.

Yes, I am sure, that the marks are not what I would change in this society. I would change the attitude or parents' ambitions towards their children that are many times unreal and do not consider the child's individuality and abilities, and remain out of reach for the child.

If only I knew how, I would try to make parents understand that many lumberjacks are happier, calmer and more fulfilled than many economists. Still more, I know many engineers that transferred to management positions and are now deprived of pleasure and personal growth and their being is being killed every day. We all know how socially productive the sad and 'unrealized' leaders really are.

No, marks have nothing to do with it.

Another thing I would change or emphasize more is the child psychologist checkup at the age of three. A real specialist can recognize a fair share of children with special needs in their early childhood. Are those checkups really performed in a proper way? How can a specialist assess a child's progress during a half-hour conversation at seven o'clock in the morning when a child is still sleepy because his mom woke him up from his dreams and with that disturbed the rhythm of the morning ritual? And then, the specialist is supposed to drag the most out of the child as fast as possible, which would help him recognize what the little one knows and is capable of doing?

How many daycare workers and teachers are familiar with the basic criteria of diagnostics for working with children with special needs? How many different diagnoses do they know at least by description? How many seminars do teachers of a first grade, who are the adults that are many times the first ones to accept a child into the school system, attend? Regarding the trend that children with a disorder are enrolled into regular school programs I think that also the education of pedagogical workers regarding this issue should be at a higher level. How far do schools and other educational institutions enable education of pedagogical workers about children that are smart enough to pass a class but are particular in their behavior?

How far can a psychologist even include himself into the work in the first grade? Can he get an idea of a child's behavior and of his maturity to enter school? How far is the parents' determination included, which can only harm a child?

And last of all—where in all of that is the role of the mother?

Today I know that I need marks and teacher's opinion to see the image of the child within social standards, which I as a mother cannot see due to my partiality. In the end, parents also raise our children for their entrance into the society and not as a permanent decoration in our living room. Society is also a competition, rivalry and noise. Institutions teach the children basics for spreading the information on life, and mothers can select schools with less noise because the children need more time to accept the noise. They need to accept it because it is part of their lives.

So, from my point of view, school reports are the right thing, but only within the child's immediate environment, the one that is held together by the marks. A person that never spent one afternoon without the presence of parents or never went to a parent-teacher meeting with a parent doesn't know how and may not evaluate a child based on his marks. A school report provides far too little information for such a person, regardless of how many books on children with special needs that person had read. Such a person can love a child but will not receive the marks from me.

Anyway, the state protects any child in such a way that enables the parents to think about such decisions independently and decide for ourselves. This is the right way and I want it to stay like that.

I believe that my first reaction on whether to show the report to the relatives or not was the right one. Regardless of whether they understood my reasons or not. With children with special needs the opinion of the society comes second and I knew that even before my learning path of child's schooling started.

One responsibility of a mother is also to protect the child but she has to gradually remove the shield and prepare the child for life as much as possible, regardless of the child's individuality.

The first one who told me that was a father of a child with Down's syndrome. And he was right. However, the path to the child's independence might sometimes be longer and with more curves for some children.

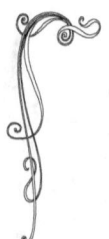

Two Sons, One Mother

I have two sons but I mostly write about my younger one. It is a fact that they are both marvelous and that I am proud of both of them equally every single moment. However, I also believe that the individualities of my younger son influenced our family life, including my older son. Even though he is twenty months older, he surely felt the difference I had made between them even though I love and respect them both equally. I tried to act in such a way that the older one would be minimally deprived of socializing with peers and socializing in general due to the individualities of the younger son. The boys got along very well ever since they were little and I never had any real problems regarding jealousy or anything like that. I was really careful not to transfer my responsibilities to my older son in the sense of watching over his brother and similar, however, the older son developed this protective, mature relationship with his younger brother when he was little already.

In the first grade at the previous school, prior to our move to Medvode, my older son had a schoolmate with Autism and the teacher at that time taught the whole class how to accept this difference. This was a relief for me because the older son accepted all our individualities during the moment of my search for answers and he took them for something completely normal. He accepted the talk on differences very maturely, but still I explained to him that he should consider the difference like a person's characteristic by which we are all different, and not like a problem or a disease.

"Sometimes I squint, you are light-tanned and you have to wear shirts when exposed to the sun, and your brother exposes feelings to strangers too intensely. I want to teach your brother not to hug everyone he trusts just like I have to protect your skin from getting burned. When I am anxious and surrounded by people, I squint, and this behavior of mine bothers me; similarly, your brother is upset because he feels like he doesn't have many friends. But we love each other regardless of our skin color, shape of eyes or behavioral individualities."

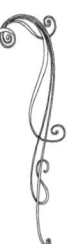

We spent a lot of time talking about his brother's individuality and soon he accepted everything that was said, especially when he realized his brother was calming down. There was a problem only during the period when his brother was in the first grade, when we first discovered the problem. During this period, when the younger child was looking for shelter with his older brother due to mutilated feeling of security it influenced the friends of the older son.

In the moments of distress the younger son many times went into the classroom of the older son for shelter. True, it was still in the lower grade and there were no marks but it for sure wasn't pleasant for him to see his younger brother at the door running into the classroom during the math lesson and hiding under his desk. The ten-year-old was bothered by emotional encounters in the hallway or in the school dining area, but felt utterly uncomfortable when his brother hugged or kissed teenagers, older than both of them, on the cheeks.

Yes, the younger child found many friends among much younger or much older children than him. He led the younger ones and understood them at their level of socialization, and had older ones for shelter. It bothered my older son more and more.

All of that influenced my decision on transferring the child. We must love each other but it is even more important that I respect both of my children. I understand that the behavior of a child with special needs bothers a teenager when trying to fit into society that is why it was even more important to me to enable both of them stress-free entrance into school and communication with peers because hanging out with schoolmates and friends is just as demanding for one as for the other. We need to adjust our limitations according to each other and not destroy or harm the formation of one's being while doing that and I wanted to be as fair as possible in this issue.

To maintain and respect the differences and individualities on each level was a task I was hardly able to handle. The solution to this task was only in talks that is why we were talking about our individualities every time any of the children brought up this subject and there was a period when we talked about it every single day.

At first, I may have demanded too much from them because they were really smart and I wanted society to finally see how well-read they were. They are still little boys, healthy and smart who sometimes forget or lose their toys in their distraction. If life were a bit more intense when we were moving to the new house I am sure they would even lose their heads. The organization level of their work environment was such that only a truly calm person could handle. And because I am only human it used to rumble in our house.

"Mommy, solve the problem constructively, don't get mad at us!" my younger son wisely taught me one night while I was nagging. His bold words took my breath away.

I immediately sent both of my boys to bed and after I had read a story I asked them:

"Well boys, what do you suggest? What is the solution for having all the notebooks in your schoolbags, pencils and crayons cleared up and pajamas folded under your pillows?"

"Oh, mom, you have a university degree, you will come up with something, you know your way around," my older son replied in a slightly patronizing manner. "Just don't complicate and everything will be all right. You'll see."

I still don't know whether he was provoking or not but I do know that it worked. When they fell asleep I sat behind the computer and wrote down a list of chores I demanded from them each day. I put dates at the top and in the middle there

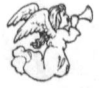

was room for ticks.

Cut commands, make them simple and do not complicate—that was my motto. That was the first real step towards the world of simple commands, equally demanding for both of them.

The next day I showed them the chart and put it on the closet door.

A miracle happened—the chart worked! Both of my sons, the older and the younger one, accepted the list and the ritual of ticks and crosses became our daily evening ritual. They both look forward to the ticks and I no longer have to yell.

Yes, we were all learning the new steps.

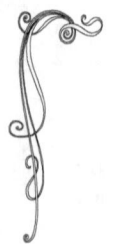

Individuality Can Also Be an Advantage

The more I got to know the individuality of my son, the easier it was for me to include it into our daily routine; soon I realized it could also be an advantage in life.

The first advantage that was very welcome was thoroughness.

When my son understood what I wanted from him he did exactly that. I wasn't allowed to say that he should 'drink the whole lake', I knew that much, but the tasks that he was able to complete he completed with an extraordinary thoroughness and care. All he understood, he completed.

If I ordered him to stand still until I say otherwise, he stood there and I could be sure that he would stand there so I was able to count on him. If I told him to wipe the table he wiped it clean and the table was dry at the end and the work perfectly done. There was no carelessness, self-adjustment of rules or inconsistency. What I required he fulfilled. Thoroughness is a characteristic that anyone can use in life and I was proud my son had it.

The next characteristic that I discover with him in everyday life is his honesty. In spite of his age and the influence from society he does not have opportunism or self-interest in himself. He would always tell me the truth (even if he didn't benefit from it) and be honest to everyone around him. Chocolate will be divided to equal chunks and so will his attentiveness. He puts himself into the shoes of others and animals and relives a moment, an event or a feeling. When he heard that a chocolate could shorten the dog's life for one year he carefully watched over her not to steal a single peace. He is very

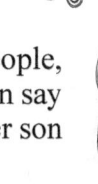

unrelenting in his kindness, his sense for animals and people, and his honesty. If a doctor ever prescribes me a diet I can say goodbye to all the culinary delights forever if my younger son takes care of me.

His third and very useful advantage is his ability to negotiate. One of the first things I did in my life when first faced with the diagnosis was that I 'classified commands into three baskets'.

The red basket had relatively few commands; however, they were all related to safety and survival and were thus strict, clear and unchangeable. This basket provided safety.

The green basket also contained only few commands and they were such that I didn't care whether the child obeyed them or not. I was willing to loosen up if necessary and if he was able to convince me with arguments that the work wasn't really necessary. Each time I would of course tell him the reason why I changed my mind and each time we would talk about it.

The biggest was and still is the orange basket. It contains most of our everyday life. The child has his obligations that he needs to fulfill. When he fights any of those obligations (and there is surprisingly only little fight) we sit and talk about a compromise that is acceptable to both of us.

For example:

For lunch I always demand from him to eat some of the vegetables.

The boy fights: "Mom, today I don't want to eat zucchini."

"Look son, I made zucchini for lunch and I want you to eat all of them. You do not want to eat even one piece. A compromise is that you eat half. Do you agree that we both let go a little and you mix half of zucchini into the potatoes and eat that mix so that we are both satisfied?"

"Ok mom, I will measure the exact half. Is that ok?"

Such compromise helps both of us. For me, they help me

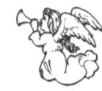

differentiate between what is really necessary and what isn't and for the child because I don't agitate him for every little thing but I still have my authority.

The most important thing and most certainly no the last one I learned from my son is unconditional love that he expresses every single moment. In our family we love each other that is why many times we teach each other and even criticize each other in good faith. My younger son is the master of this issue because he loves without criticism. When he loves he loves and accepts everything about you unconditionally.

When I am angry, sad or helpless, he crawls to me and says: "I love you when you are sad, also."

When the older son does something stupid, something utterly inappropriate, the younger one hugs him and says: "Don't worry, you are the best brother in the world."

In my lonely moments I feel like I have an ally that accepts me for what I am all the time. It is such a priceless feeling, each of us needs it and many do not know how to give it!

From my little teacher we all learn to accept and love unconditionally.

To love unconditionally. This is a characteristic that puts everything else into shade. And this is my child's characteristic.

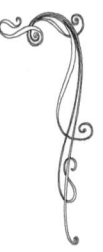

Noise and Music

Many times I mentioned my child's response to noise. I don't think I can find another thing or occurrence that would have such a strong disturbing impact on him. Every time I think about visiting a social event or a meeting I think about the influence of all the sudden vibrations or noise on my son. With each similar event I think about how to prepare the child for such disturbing stimuli.

Music has a totally different impact.

Ever since he was little he has had the perfect sense for rhythm and movement and listens to a wide spectrum of music. Every time he has a chance he comes up to the CD player and selects a song. He listens to it with feeling, with full attention. When his older brother is not around he goes to the middle of the room, closes his eyes and surrenders to the movement. I cannot say it is dancing because his movement is surrendered to the waves of music that sometimes reminds me to a soft stream of a clear creek that transforms with his distinct movement of his whole body into slow whirl of a deep pool and then calms down into the embrace of the sun. And when he hugs the sun with the wings of a butterfly he sits in his movements on the most tender flower on the lawn. This expression of his illustrates the clarity of the child's soul. With this feeling of tenderness in music that same child greets a flower in the meadow, a lion at the zoo and a teacher at school with a soft voice. Everything he touches with his gracefulness is immediately filled with love and warmth.

I've loved music ever since I can remember and in high school I loved going to the expressive dance school but one cannot teach a child what my son expresses with his motion.

67

Dance, motion and rhythm were put into his crib. In every activity that he participated, all the mentors, daycare teachers and teaches, all that felt his love for music, told me to enroll him into music school.

The last year of his pre-school period I enrolled him into an excellent private music school that he attended until the performances started and until the moment that he had to learn rigid scales. With the rigid rules of performances his learning in music school ended. Why?

Society demands performances. Mommies and daddies want to see their children perform on stage. Even better, when the whole world and the whole family see their (maybe even) talented boy. Children must stand in line, must go on stage, must stand there in line and on mentor's mark show what the teachers decided they knew best.

When a child is not performing under pressure and in a way that is so very strict, only then can he show what he is capable of.

It took my younger son years to get ready for his first performance. Performing, playing and reciting in front of a crowd were taboo until recently. As early as daycare it was hard to get him to cooperate at rehearsal within the limits of strict rules of group performance. The daycare teachers had their hands full to make him obey the rules at the rehearsals. When it was time to perform he wouldn't get on the stage. Even when only the closest families were in the audience my child was numb with fear and stage fright to the extent that a performance meant nothing but fear and restlessness and also outbursts which numbed the performance of other children, too.

I saw my child for the first time completely relaxed performing at the final production in the second grade. Congratulations to the teacher who was able to achieve that.

That performance is another milestone in our lives.

Since that performance I have been constantly looking for a dance school with open rules. I am not familiar with economy of dance and music schools but I sincerely wish to find a teacher that would offer parents with no ambitions to teach their children expressive dance. I wish that every child would have the possibility to express his feelings in a way closest to him. For a child that cannot stand the noise and thus doesn't participate in sports games in gyms where noise is omnipresent, can hardly express his distress and feelings through sports, it would be nice if I could direct him into music. Music and sports clear the soul and fill it with peace and love and this is what every child and every adult needs sooner or later.

Is there a teacher with love for children great enough that would teach children who do not tolerate strict rules and noise? I think it would be challenge for many experts.

I live to see the day when I will meet a person that is willing to step out of the world of strict society standards. I would like to meet people who would like to nourish natural characteristics in their children like the students and their mentors taught my younger child to swim when he was four months old knowing that in life without society limitations anything is possible.

Like all natural beings the parents develop and learn. And just like the cliché of a child learning how to swim in late daycare period was shattered I hope that one day there will be a person who will let a six-year-old with behavioral limitations at a level of a three-year-old express his feelings while dancing with qualities and at a level of a talented dancer but without strict requirements of ballet or hip hop.

I wish for a spontaneous, open, accepting society at all levels of sporting and cultural expression. Only time will tell how such a process is evaluated.

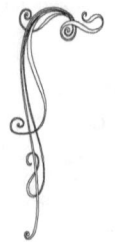

Parent-Teacher Meeting Two Years Later

It was a hot summer day. I left work an hour earlier Than usual because an evaluation of my child's progress with school representatives was scheduled at Topol school. To say it differently, the school invited me to a meeting at the end of the school year with all the people that were intensely working with my child. Another parent-teacher meeting...

It was a day like many others. I sat in the overheated car, let the windows down and played some music. Like a thousand times before I checked my watch and realized I was only going to be a couple of minutes late. It's all right. Both of the boys are still at school, the older one has tennis lessons after school and I can deal with parent-teacher meeting for the younger one in peace. The way to school was clear, traffic was low. I entered the building with music in my heart and I overheard a conversation in the classroom. I listened closely. My son was talking to the school manager. It had to be some serious conversation, something to do with crayons. The tone of the conversation was calm. I repressed my motherly concern and followed the teacher into the library. My son was finishing the third grade. I was proud of him.

All four sat at the table at the school library: Erika on my left, teacher Polona opposite me, and Lovro on my right. The teacher opened the meeting almost too formally, but her tone did not confuse me. I'd grown to love her a long time ago. With her gracefulness and authority and in a very warm way she was able to make my son sit still for 45 minutes behind his desk and participate in the lessons from the first day on. She is the teacher that gained so much trust with my son that he remained calm even in the most critical situations, like for

70

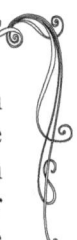

example a month ago when he unfortunately stepped between the radiator ribs and they were not able to pull his leg from the trapped position she was able to prepare him for a situation in which the janitor would most probably have to cut the radiator with a noisy saw and my son remained calm even though he anticipated the noise. This is a woman that succeeded during one school year in a warm and soft manner to make my son fulfill his obligations. I trusted her more than anyone.

"What was going on in the classroom when I arrived? I heard such serious conversation," I asked her.

"Well, it was basically a nice event. A girl told your son that she would not lend him her crayons because she doesn't want the crayons to be broken. So he calmly went to the principal and asked her what it actually meant—that she is looking after her crayons or that she thinks he breaks everything?"

"My child did not burst out but calmly asked for someone's opinion???"

Then I was finally relieved. Erika, specialist teacher that works with my son, and teacher Polona were listing examples when my son remained calm in similar situations. I was listening to them but in my mind I was reliving the previous school year at the previous school when it was a miracle if that same child was able to sit through the whole lesson at the desk. I remember he had to be removed from the classroom forcefully a few times for starting to rage at other children.

"He almost doesn't use his corner anymore. He only stretches rubber a little when he is upset but he calms down," Lovro continued.

Lovro is the companion to my child and an assistant at after-school care. Curly hair, tall, and slender young man, seemingly almost too young for such difficult role. Fresh from the faculty he's got everything my child needs: peace, self-confidence, work habits, patience, maturity and love for children. Only today I know how desperately I needed a calm approach of a mature man when working with my child to complement the picture of loving female figures in my son's life. Ever since Lovro came to our lives my son became a little man that learned from a calm, mature, balanced person in a manly way, unknown to me. I was not able to give that feeling to him and I never would be regardless of all the read books. Thank you, Lovro.

The meeting continued with the evaluation and with the report of what my son can do and what my son knows. Everything I heard I already knew. The difference was that a group of people who were working with my child on daily basis were describing my son's abilities to me. It was the first time that I didn't do the talking of how smart and creative he was. It wasn't me, persuading other people how extremely talented he was in narrating and that he is good at logical thinking. The teacher and the specialist teacher told me that this child, who was a year ago labeled as disturbing at a playground, even as a fool, was the only one that solved the test at the republic competition without a single mistake and that he was going to receive a special award for it. When they asked me whether I allowed them to nominate him for program for talented pupils I was wiping my tears of gratefulness and nodding my head because I just wasn't able to talk anymore.

A smart, calm and much more mature child ended his third year of elementary school. At the graduation ceremony I was so proud I wanted to dance and cheer out loud. Proudly I complimented his effort and awards, grateful to life for having hope again for the child to finish elementary school and be ready for entrance into society, into life.

I was grateful to that cuckoo in the forest.

After the award ceremony a snack was organized for the pupils at the Gostišče ob Ločnici guesthouse. Two children from the ninth grade were saying goodbye and their parents invited all of the participants to a picnic. I agreed to attend the picnic with both of my boys, but with some fear. Deep inside, the fear of noisy events was still very present. But it was nice.

72

The children played at the football playground and the parents chatted with the school staff. Just as I was talking to the school principle, I noticed on the other side of the meadow that there was a quarrel between two children—and one of them was my younger son. At one point my child swiftly turned away from the others, went to the edge of the forest and stared at a tree. Without going closer I could tell he was very angry.

"What is going to happen, where did he go?" I jumped.

"He is angry so he went to calm down," Erika, the special teacher who works with him, explained.

I was about to run over there to calm him down but she stopped me.

"Don't be afraid, nothing is going to happen. Everything will be alright," she said.

At that moment, my older son and a group of peers approached his brother, he put his hand on his shoulder and they left together to kick ball into the goal.

The tears veiled my sight. I watched the boys play and thought of the past. I saw all the past battles at the playgrounds, heard all the screams and yells that we so many times experienced. At that moment I relived so many unjust moments we experienced together, but conquered them and remained together, strong and united in love. Then I immediately realized that all the effort was not in vain. We won. We defeated the clichés and the limitations and learned many truths in life. We remained connected and warm, strong in our recognitions and strong in our steps towards learning life.

And what is worth the most—we conquered fear.

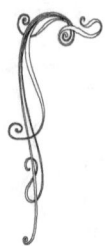

Asperger and I

He is a great man, this Asperger. I heard his name two and a half years ago. I wasn't aware of what kind of school was awaiting me. I even don't know what kind of surprise this man is preparing for me tomorrow maybe. All I feel towards him is my sincere gratefulness. I am grateful for him teaching the experts how to teach us, mothers, to hear and understand our children. I am grateful for his published literature so that my reasoning has support for understanding the behavior of society towards my child and that he was by my side when I was looking for answers to the most difficult questions.

There was a period when we were together in my mind day and night. Even though I've been living a happy and divorced life for quite a while I did not want to lean on my ex-husband on my path of searching because I wasn't able to coordinate such a hard test with a demanding relationship after the divorce. I was informing my ex-husband regularly on all the procedures and tests correctly, but I did not share my feelings with him as I had enough of my own tests and questions. In those moments, I desperately needed some support but not in the form of plain and long questioning and requests for explanations. That is why Mr. Asperger was always closer to me than the child's father. Nevertheless, I think that the latter would most definitely describe his experience of our child's individuality in a different way.

During this period I accepted Mr. Asperger subconsciously, sometimes like a personal friend and in a certain period he was even some kind of partner as together we were chasing all the intruders and wise guys away, all those people that were occupying me and asking too many questions. He was by my side though my whole process of searching myself and my being and many times he understood that many of evenings I did not need another new question. Then we went to the forest. We walked the desolated paths where I demanded answers harshly, sometimes even stubbornly, without being aware of it. However, whenever I demanded something from him, he would hide. I would call after him, beg him, scream to come back, but he wouldn't. He would leave me on the path full of fear and the distress in me only grew. Then I subconsciously and forcefully looked for answers to the most egoistic questions.

"Why is this happening to me, precisely?"

"Why does life demand so much strength from me?"

"Why do I have to repress all my expectations regarding the child?"

No, I never wanted or expected my children to become respected, highly recognized gentlemen in high places. I know too many unhappy people fastened in their own restraints that perform their very respectable jobs as managers, lawyers and doctors with an empty, sad, and unfulfilled look and each moment their faces show how very far they actually are from their own real being. I was never ambitious regarding my sons. But elementary school—this is the basis! Without elementary school there is no elementary education and even a very smart person should have some basics, not just on paper. The elementary school teaches the basis for life and our way of living requires this basis.

All those questions pushed me down the paths that led to my stump. My companion knew everything that was happening to me very well. He understood my distress, my loneliness in all the troubles a day brings. He was my support until the very moment I accepted my role, the lesson I had to learn. To embrace and grow to love every single challenge I experienced—that was a moment of personal victory that brought back my pride. When I left the forest an hour or two later with self-confidence my teacher joined me again with a smile on his face.

"Have you realized that all of that is not happening to you?"

He did not need an answer; he was able to read it from my face, from my calm eyes and smile, ready for new challenges.

My teacher and my leader was with me all the time. Sometimes he had pity on me and provided an answer when I least expected one and he always cheered me up in my revelation that this is all part of the maturity given to me by life. Sometimes, when I needed him the most and I tamely closed my weary eyes, helpless, he hugged me, squeezed me and with a soft velvet voice said: "I believe in you, girl, you can do it!"

Now when I'm writing this book I look back and realize that he taught me how to live. He taught me how to accept a moment just as it is. Planning and organizing work should remain at work. At home, all I want is peace, love and laughter and the joy of the moment that I share open-heartedly with my sons. When any of us put our tired heads into another one's lap and feel a calm hand lovingly curling a lock of hair we all love, we know that we have everything that a person can truly have in his life. Precious feeling of love and acceptance is the supreme award for the lessons we all learned.

Yes, my precious teacher, by your merit I allow anything. There was a time when I didn't know my son, that is why I am totally aware that anything is possible and that I don't know anyone. Today I do not judge anymore. I don't judge anyone, not even those who want to hurt me on purpose. Their desire is a part of them and my desire is to accept them the way they are with everything they do or express. What they think—no, I don't know that and I don't want to know it. I just want to know and feel how they treat me now, what they express in their communication with me and if they want to be a part of my story.

76

Thank you, Mr. Asperger. Thank you for this lesson, thank you for the school I graduated from with you by my side. Today, I am ready for the next level. I know there will be a number of new lessons. But the fear is gone.

Thank you for all the wonderful people that stood by my side and thank you for all the moments of revelation; those are truly priceless.

And thank you, life, for such marvelous children.

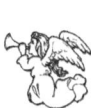

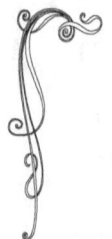

In Short—How to Accept the Tough School of Life

When I was looking for the answers, I found only a very few life stories with similar experience about children with special needs and their mothers. The experts told me to stay away from forums and soon I agreed with them because know-it-alls can write anything under their nickname and a hurt mother can be an easy target for being led into the total opposite direction. Down's syndrome, Asperger's syndrome, autism—all of those individualities are very specific and today I understand why I received so little directions for life from the experts. Behavior and sensitivity are different for each child and even more different is the child's reaction to numerous daily life events. There is really not much written about parent experience.

When a colleague invited me home to his warm family circle that lives a quality life with a child with Down's syndrome, I knew our children were different. But the words of that child's parents were similar to those I write here. Let me sum up a few of their thoughts that led me though this whole learning period.

I received approximately such advices:

1. First, listen to yourself. Nobody knows your child like you do, so in spite of things you didn't know and you learned from strangers don't think that an expert that guided you for a month or two knows your child better than you do. Re-establish the trust in your motherhood and be supportive of the child regardless of the tests ahead of you.

2. Put yourself and your needs to the same level as the child. If you are 'put together' your child will feel it and in that one hour you spend with him he will share more with you than

if you were with him all the time but totally absent-minded. Recreation, company or an hour in the forest will clean your valves to such extent that you can offer your child much more than otherwise.

3. Accept. Accept your child's individuality as soon as possible. The longer you put it off the longer you will suffer and it will be harder for you and your child. Your child needs you and by accepting his individuality you will be closer to him and you will benefit from it.

4. Make selection of your friends. Once your curtain is revealed and your sight of your life is clear many 'friends' will leave. Don't feel sad because apparently they cannot handle the individuality. True ones will come, those who can accept the individuality and will stand by your side without expressing their supremacy. Those are the only appropriate people for you and your child.

5. Above all—don't blame yourself. Be proud that the angels trusted you with such special child. They know that you are a great mother who can stand by the side of a child with special needs. They know that you are not perfect but they also believe that in spite of that, you are worthy of their trust and you have all the right to be proud of that.

6. And the most important thing of all: love yourself. Not just your child. Love yourself and be tender to yourself. Tenderness is all you and your children need.

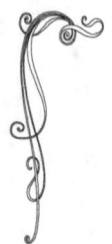

Appendix 1: Chart of Tasks for Both Children

DATE:			
ADDITIONAL:			
Help mother with the chores.			
Take care of Taja.			
Learn for fifteen minutes.			
Improve my notebook.			
EVERY DAY:			
Clean the toilet and the sink after use.			
Take laundry to the laundry room.			
Fold my pajamas under the pillow.			
What I spill I clean.			
After a meal clear the table.			
Return a book to its shelf.			
Put toys where they belong.			
Prepare the pencil case for school.			
Prepare school bag.			
Prepare gym uniform for school.			
Prepare slippers for school.			
Negative points:			
I was at school without slippers.			
I was at school without gym uniform.			

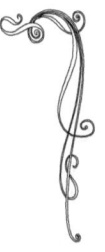

Appendix 2: Diagnosis Criteria

Diagnostic Criteria for Asperger Disorder (Gilberg and Gilberg – 1989)

1. Severe impairment in reciprocal social interaction (at least two of the following):
   - inability to interact with peers
   - lack of desire to interact with peers
   - lack of appreciation of social cues
   - socially and emotionally inappropriate behavior
2. All-absorbing narrow interest (at least one of the following)
   - exclusion of other activities
   - repetitive adherence
   - more rote than meaning
3. Imposition of routines and interests (at least one of the following)
   - on self, in aspects of life
   - on others
4. Speech and language problems (at least three of the following)
   - delayed development
   - superficially perfect expressive language
   - formal, pedantic language
   - odd prosody, peculiar voice characteristics

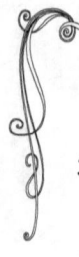

- impairment of comprehension including misinterpretations of literal/implied meanings

5. Non-verbal communication problems (at least one of the following)
   - limited use of gestures
   - clumsy/gauche body language
   - limited facial expression
   - inappropriate expression
   - peculiar, stiff gaze

6. Motor clumsiness: poor performance on neurodevelopmental examination

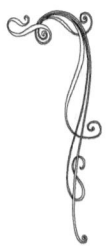

Diagnostic Criteria for Asperger Disorder (Szatmari, Bremner and Nagy – 1989)

1. Social isolation (at least two of the following):
   - no close friends
   - avoids others
   - no interest in making friends
   - a loner
2. Impaired social interaction (at least one of the following):
   - approaches others only to have own needs met
   - clumsy social approach
   - one-sided responses to peers
   - difficulty sensing feelings of others
   - indifference to the feelings of others
3. Impaired non-verbal communication (at least one of the following):
   - limited facial expressions
   - impossible to read emotions through facial expression of the child
   - inability to convey message with eyes
   - avoids looking at others
   - does not use hands to aid expression
   - large and clumsy gestures
   - infringes on other people's physical space
4. Speech and language peculiarities (at least two of the following):

83

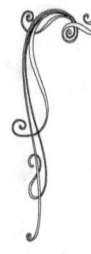

- abnormalities of inflection
- over-talkative
- non-communicative
- lack of cohesion to conversation
- idiosyncratic use of words
- repetitive patters of speech

5. Does not meet the criteria DSM-111-R for: autism

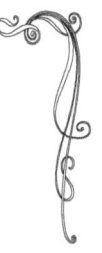

Diagnostic Criteria for Asperger Disorder
(DSM IV – 1994)

1. Qualitative impairment in social interaction (at least two of the following):

   - marked impairment in the use of multiple nonverbal behaviors such as eye-to-eye gaze, facial expression, body postures, and gestures to regulate social interaction

   - failure to develop peer relationships appropriate to developmental level

   - lack of spontaneous seeking to share enjoyment, interests, or achievements with other people (e.g., by a lack of showing, bringing, or pointing out objects of interest to other people.

   - lack of social or emotional reciprocity

2. Restricted repetitive and stereotyped patterns of behavior, interests and activities (at least one of the following):

   - encompassing preoccupation with one or more stereotyped and restricted patterns of interest that is abnormal either in intensity or focus

   - apparently inflexible adherence to specific, nonfunctional routines or rituals

   - stereotyped and repetitive motor mannerisms (e.g., hand or finger flapping or twisting, or complex whole-body movements)

   - persistent preoccupation with parts or objects

3. The disturbance causes clinically significant impairment in social, occupational, or other important areas of functioning.

4. There is no clinically significant general delay in language (e.g. single words used by age two, communicative phrases used by age three).

5. There is no clinically significant delay in cognitive development or in the development of age-appropriate self-help skills, adaptive behavior (other than in social interaction), and curiosity about the environment in childhood.

6. Criteria are not met for another specific Pervasive Developmental Disorder or Schizophrenia.

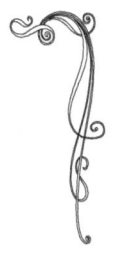

Diagnostic Criteria for Asperger Disorder (ICD- 10 – World Health Organization, 1993)

1. A lack of any clinically significant general delay in spoken or receptive language or cognitive development. Diagnosis requires that single words should have developed by two years of age or earlier and that communicative phrases be used by three years of age or earlier. Self-help skills, adaptive behavior and curiosity about the environment during the first three years should be at a level consistent with intellectual development. However, motor milestones may be somewhat delayed and motor clumsiness is usual (although not a necessary diagnostic feature). Isolated special skills, often related to abnormal preoccupations, are common, but are not required for diagnosis.

2. Qualitative abnormalities in reciprocal social interaction (at least two of the following):

   - marked impairment in the use of multiple nonverbal behaviors such as eye-to-eye gaze, facial expression, body postures, and gestures to regulate social interaction

   - failure to develop peer relationships appropriate to developmental level regardless of numerous opportunities

   - lack of social or emotional reciprocity reflected in unsuitable and extraordinary response to emotions of others or lack of behavior adjustment in regard to social context or poor integration of social, emotional and communicative behavior

   - lack of spontaneous seeking to share enjoyment, interests, or achievements with other people (e.g., by a lack of showing, bringing, or pointing out objects of interest to others.

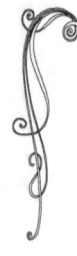

3. An unusually intense circumscribed interest or restrictive, repetitive, and stereotyped patterns of behavior, interests and activities (at least one of the following):

- encompassing preoccupation with one or more stereotyped and restricted patterns of interest that is abnormal either in intensity or focus

- apparently inflexible adherence to specific, nonfunctional routines or rituals

- stereotyped and repetitive motor mannerisms (e.g., hand or finger flapping or twisting, or complex whole-body movements)

- persistent preoccupation with parts or objects

4. The disorder is not attributable to other varieties of pervasive developmental disorder: schizotypal disorder, simple schizophrenia, obsessive-compulsive disorder, anancastic personality disorder, and disinhibited attachment disorder of childhood.

Literature

Attwood T., ' Asperger's syndrome: a guide for parents and professionals' – Radomlje: Megaton, 2007 (Slovene translation)

Attwood, A. J., Frith, V. and Hermelin (1 998) 'The understanding and use of interpersonal guesures by autistic and Down's syndrome children', Journal of Autism and Developmental Disorders 1 8,2,241 -257

Cessaroni, L. and Garber, M. (1 991) 'Exploring the experience of autism through first hand accounts'. Journal of Autism and Developmental Disorders 21 ,303-31 3

Fine, J., Bartolucci, G., Ginsberg, G. and Szatmari, P. (1 991) 'The use of intonation to communicate in Pervasive Developmental Disorders'. Journal of Child Psychology and Psychiatry 32,777-782

Gillberg, C. (1 991) 'Clinical and neurobiological aspects of Asberger Syndrome in six family studies.' In U. Frith (ed) Autism and Asberger Syndrome, Cambridge: Cambridge University Press.

Gillberg, C., Gillberg, I.C. and Staffenburg, S. (1 992) 'Siblings and parents of children with autism: A controlled population based study'. Developmental Medicine and Child Neurology 34,389-398 11 5

Szatmari, P., Archer, L., Fisman, S., Streiner, D.L. and Wilson, F. (1 995) 'Asperger's Syndrome and autism: Differences in behaviour, cognition and adaptive functioning.' Journal of the American Academy of Child and Adolescent Pschyiatry 34,1 662-1 671

Szatmari, P., Bartolucci, G. And Bremner, R. (1 989) 'Asperger's Syndrome and autism: Comparison of early history and outcome.'

Developmental Medicine and Child Neurology 31, 709-720.

WHO (1 989) Tenth Revision of the International Classification ofDisease Geneva: World Health Organization.

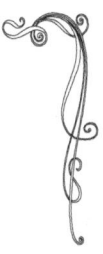

Kazalo

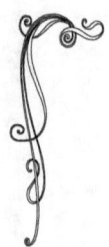

www.ingramcontent.com/pod-product-compliance
Lightning Source LLC
Chambersburg PA
CBHW071243170526
45165CB00003B/1212